IGNITE!

THE ULTIMATE GUIDE TO HOLISTIC WEIGHT LOSS,
FEELING CONFIDENT IN YOUR OWN BODY,
AND UNLOCKING YOUR FULL POTENTIAL

Joel Evan

Edited by Melissa Ryan

Formatted by Sophie Hanks

Table of Content

Introduction

6.8%

I never wanted to be a "weight loss coach." Hell, I never even had weight problems in my life so what would compel me to care enough to write a book about it? The answer is trifold. First, my childhood was plagued by health issues that were accepted as 'normal.' But, when I reached adulthood and saw some of my dearest loved ones suffering from a variety of physical ailments, I could not accept their suffering as 'normal' so I vowed to do as much as possible to help them get better. Second, in my quest to improve my own health and to help my loved ones, I have amassed a vast education in holistic and alternative medicine that I feel compelled to share with others. Third, I've always dreamt of being a part of something bigger than myself, and I have a passion to lessen human suffering and disease so that people can reach the highest versions of themselves.

What does all of this have to do with losing weight? The answer is – everything! My journey and my education have made it clear to me that excess weight is as much a symptom of underlying physical and psychological health issues as it is a cause of those problems. This means that losing weight doesn't necessarily make you healthy. Instead, getting mentally and physically healthy will enable you to lose weight.

I can imagine the ripple effect that it will create in the world if my work and my words can improve even just one person's quality of life. If I can help someone become more aligned with their truth so that they end up healthy, vibrant, and full of energy and confidence and their weight is no longer holding them back from unlocking their full potential, then the effort of writing this book is well worth it.

Knowing this and wanting to share this is what drives me. This is my inspiration for writing this book. This is what ignites my passion!

My passion has been further fueled by some startling research into the metabolic health of Americans. Metabolic health is a term used to describe how well we generate and process energy in the body. Clinically speaking, it is measured by five markers: blood sugar, triglycerides, high-density lipoprotein (HDL), cholesterol, and waist circumference. Good metabolic health means that those numbers are all at optimal levels – without medication. Yet, a 2019 publication reported that only 12% of Americans were metabolically healthy — defined as having no criteria of metabolic syndrome while free of medications. Then a 2022 study reported that only 6.8% of Americans had "optimal" levels of metabolic health markers. It is worth repeating – only 6.8% of Americans are considered metabolically healthy. That's a travesty!

It is also a danger. Poor metabolic health not only makes it difficult to maintain a healthy weight, it also raises the risk for developing all the diseases that come with unhealthy weight - diabetes, insulin resistance, Alzheimer's disease, atherosclerosis, heart problems, high blood pressure, low energy, fatigue, and mood issues such as depression.

So, although I have not struggled with weight problems, I come to this from a place of empathy and understanding since I have struggled with health issues. Growing up, I was not particularly healthy. I suffered from regular earaches and colds and was seemingly always on penicillin to kill those infections. Also, when I was ten years old, my parents noticed that I had this weird lump on the inner part of my left thigh. They thought it was just a contusion from a baseball hitting me, but the bump never disappeared. After taking me to the hospital for X-rays, the doctors (all practitioners of strictly Western medicine) confirmed that it was an "abnormal bone growth." We were told, "Not to worry, we'll just go in and chisel it off and sew Joel backup." But there was no explanation as to why this had occurred. "Things like this just happen…" is what the doctors told my mom. Who can relate?

Can you also relate to my childhood diet? I grew up on a diet of processed food and artificial flavors. My daily lunch through grade school and most of high school was a peanut butter sandwich on white bread, a Capri-Sun, and some kind of dessert such as a Nutter Butter, a Hostess cupcake, a fruit rollup, etc. And when I came home from school every day, I was allowed one soda daily. For dinner, I never ate anything green and mostly ate chicken marinated in processed Teriyaki glaze or pasta with Prego sauce. A healthy breakfast for me was Cheerios versus Cinnamon Toast Crunch. Looking back at my childhood diet, it's no wonder why I was sick and suffered from these illnesses. I was slowly being poisoned by toxic foods that created imbalances in my body.

Despite this – or because of this – I was very interested in exercise and physical fitness growing up. When I turned 18 years old, I was very confused about my place in the world, as I'm sure most teenagers are in their life. I was asking myself, "Who am I?" Am I a jock? Am I a nerd? Where do I fit in best in society? How do people view me? One thing I knew for certain was that I wanted more girls to like me and be attracted to me. My good friend Sean O'Keefe was a high school football player and had transformed his body through weight lifting. I thought lifting weights could be a great way for girls to notice me more and maybe transform my identity. So, I started lifting weights, and I loved it. My dad bought me a subscription to Muscle & Fitness magazine that I probably had for over three years. I geeked out on all the bodybuilders such as Flex Wheeler, Jay Cutler, Ronnie Coleman, and Dorian Yates. I would copy their workout plans and replicate whatever they were doing in the gym. I started taking supplements and eating better so that I could get bigger and more muscular.

Looking back, this was one of the most pivotal things I did in my life. By adding regular exercise to my life, I did two things: 1. I learned how to eat better to fuel my body, and 2. I unknowingly built the habits that would later cement my lifetime passion for fitness and good health. Also, instead of not knowing my place in the world, my identity became, "I go to the gym." For me, not working out six days a week actually felt weird.

I also started doing martial arts because I wanted to be more than just physically strong. I wanted the full package - improvement of mind, body, and soul. Six years later, I got my black belt in a street self-defense art known as Kajukenbo under Professor David Amiccuci. He might not be well known in terms of fame, but he is probably one of the greatest and most skilled martial artists of our time. He taught me the importance of having a bulletproof mindset and the determination to never give up. He also helped me cultivate a growth mindset and an eagerness to always want to learn more. I am forever grateful because that never-quit and never-stop-learning mindset is infused in everything I do today.

By 25 years old, though, I realized that I still did not know exactly what I wanted to do with my life. I knew I wanted to help people, and I knew I wanted to do something with my mind and body. My father, a police officer, suggested I go into law enforcement like him. My grandfather also was a police officer for the San Francisco Police Department in the 1950's-70's. I had thought that I didn't want to be like my dad and grandfather, that I wanted to be something even 'better.' Nonetheless, I was tired of living at home with my parents, and I thought it might be a good career move for me. So, I became a police officer with the Oakland Police Department – a job I proudly did for six years and then transferred to the San Francisco Police Department for almost nine years, until doing what I do now.

As much as I loved helping people through my law enforcement career, it was the birth of my first son, my mom being diagnosed with breast cancer, and watching my mother-in-law suffer from chronic health issues that made me want to change careers. I realized I had garnered all of this Western-style health knowledge throughout the years, but I was unable to help the people closest to me. That made me sad and angry. My first son suffered from gut issues like candida yeast overgrowth, experienced symptoms similar to PANS/PANDAS, and suffered from other neuro/cognitive issues. I was unwilling to accept that my son or others would suffer and go through some of the same issues that crippled me as a child. I wanted to learn how to get people better from a root-cause standpoint. It was clear to me that the Western model of medicine was not getting anyone better and was simply masking symptoms with pills.

Although I wanted to help my loved ones, I knew I couldn't go back to school and get a doctorate in naturopathy because I now had two kids and a family to support. But, I also knew that I was destined to be able to do more for them so I invested in multiple life and holistic health coaching certifications in order to learn from some of the best alternative health minds in the world. Then, at the end of 2019, I launched an alternative health podcast called The Hacked Life podcast. This became an amazing pathway that allowed me to connect with the best and brightest experts in the health and mindset world.

From there, my passion and my knowledge grew exponentially. This enabled me to start my health coaching business at the top of 2021. I focused my health coaching on weight loss because I felt that it was such a huge problem and that many weight loss gurus were making it too complicated for the average, hard-working professional to stay consistent and be successful long-term. I also felt that there were critical natural-health principles, such as the importance of a liver detox, that were not being discussed in the metabolic health world and were only being discussed in natural health circles.

For most busy professionals I work with, counting calories and macros and hitting the gym six days a week is just impractical. They have mortgages, kids, family responsibilities, overtime, shift-work, and the pace of life sweeps them away. But I knew there was a way to get impactful results despite all that other noise because I had done it myself. I've been a husband and dad for over eight years, had a side business and a mega podcast, worked 60-hour weeks in my normal job for over six years, figured out alternative ways of fitting exercise into my hectic life, and I still was able to maintain peak and optimal health. I knew if it was possible for me, given my huge workload and stresses, then it could be possible for other busy professionals. With that conviction in mind, my desire grew exponentially to teach the principles of mindset, nutrition, detox, exercise, and mastery to others so that they can get healthy and lose weight.

Then, in October of 2021, the San Francisco Police Department and I parted ways, and I went full bore into my health coaching business. In my first year, I helped over 80 people lose weight (on average, 20 lbs or more) and keep it off. The reason my coaching works so well is that it's not a "lose weight quick" scheme or some type of crash diet. I'm teaching a lifestyle. I'm teaching principles of health. It's not outcome-based like many of these crash diets – it's process based. When you understand the principles and the processes of health, you become a master of yourself. You know how to get better and retune yourself even if you come out of balance now and then or slip up on nutrition (which is bound to happen with anyone). The key is, can you come back, reorient yourself, retune into whom you say you are, and continue to live the highest version of yourself? I hope this book helps you to answer 'yes' to this question.

So, thank you for picking up this book. I'm excited for you to change your life. This book is not just a "weight loss book." It is a guide book - a handbook - to a newer, healthier way of living. It's a change of identity. It's a change of mind and a change of heart. The same principles that I teach in this book will not only change your health for the better, they also will help you to become a better spouse, brother/sister, leader, employee, boss/CEO, etc.

Let's get started making the changes that will allow you to shed both the figurative and the literal weight from your life! Let's ignite your passion and change your life!

Now let's go!!!!

Chapter 1

Mindset

Mindset

The discipline to stay disciplined is a discipline very few can master

-Bedros Keulian

Everyone knows that weight loss happens when we stay consistent with eating right and exercising. Right? But, if it were that simple, I would not have clients and you would not be reading this book. So, what then is the reason that weight loss – and maintaining that weight loss – is so hard? The answer is multifactorial, but it truly comes down to mindset.

To this end, anytime I start working with clients that want to get healthy and lose weight, the very first thing I start working on is their minds. Why? Shouldn't we focus on exercise and eating less, Joel? Well, if that were true, all of you would be successful by now, right? One of the biggest reasons my clients weren't previously successful in life or in their long-term weight loss comes down to two things: consistency and commitment.

Certainly, it is important to ask questions such as: What is the right nutrition plan for me? What should I eat and not eat? What exercise program will work for me? But, I have found that getting the right answers to those questions does not matter without the discipline to stay motivated over the course of time. Therefore, the more important questions are:

How do we attain this level of discipline?
How do we make this level of discipline feel effortless and not such a struggle so we can maintain it long-term?

It all comes down to cultivating the right mindset, mastering your beliefs, managing your expectations, and understanding motivation so that it works for you, not against you. Let's dive in.

What is the Right Mindset for Losing Weight?

Without this abiding trust, the home is but a dwelling place built on the foundations of shifting sands. Faith is the bond that perpetuates human understanding and friendship.

-Dr. Thurman Fleet

Two things are imperative for establishing a solid foundation for your weight loss journey: faith and a growth mindset.

First, you must have faith that you're going to succeed. You must believe that things will work out even though you can't see the finish line - even when the end goal is far, far away. What if you're someone that has to lose 100 lbs and you find out that it can take up to two years to lose that amount of weight? Two years from now is so far away, and many of us are living day to day. We're not even sure how our week is going to go. So, imagine how difficult it would be to plan for a whole year or two from now and actually believe that you'll reach that goal weight.

Maintaining that belief and not wavering from that goal is difficult, but it is not impossible. Since it is difficult, so many of us have been in that place where we've lost some weight and then plateaued. Then we start going back into old beliefs and old ideas such as "I'm not good enough," or "I just have a slow metabolism," or "Why does this always happen to me?" Doubt, fear, and lack of faith creep into our lives, and we move backward. The progress we've made feels all for nothing, and that brief moment of motivation and goodwill disappears, and we slip back into old routines.

When you lose faith in life like this, it's like being on a boat without a rudder. The waves of life crash your boat and take you wherever the waves of life want to take you. This lack of faith translates into a lack of mental, physical and spiritual satisfaction. When you find yourself adrift like this, you can take back control by asking yourself, "What have you ever learned from success?" Most of us have learned nothing from success because success means that it all worked out. It's the injuries, the pain, and the tough lessons that taught us to grow and get better, and, with that wisdom, we've become stronger and more resilient. In other words, remind yourself to have the faith that your setback can turn into triumph.

One of the greatest healers I've ever had the chance to be around, Dr. Pete Goldman (who's gotten people better from multiple autoimmune diseases and endometriosis, gotten people off liver transplant lists, and helped multiple athletes and professional fighters recover from what doctors said were career-ending injuries) told me, "Without faith, there is no cure." The same is true for weight loss or success in general in life. If you lack faith, you will never get better.

From a metaphysical standpoint, the more you become a master over fear, anxiety, hatred, resentment, jealousy and selfishness, the more you come into harmony with your higher self and what you were meant to accomplish. You become strengthened physically, mentally, and spiritually. The problem for many of you, though, is that you don't realize how close you are to such a breakthrough. Whether you realize it or not, you're actually on the path to exponential growth.

Exponential Growth Curve

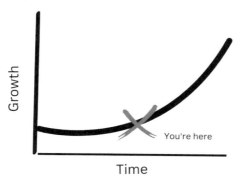

Look at where the "X" is on the Exponential Growth Curve graph below. That's about where many of us are when we start our journey. We add some new habits and maybe implement a new diet or a new workout routine, and then, all of a sudden, something happens. We look at the graph and think, "Holy sh*t! It looks like I've accomplished nothing; I'm still more or less where I started. We also look at it and say, "Sh*t! That mountain looks tough and steep to climb! I'm scared. I don't think I can do this. I'm just going to give up." And so, this cycle continues. But what if, instead, we look at the graph and see that moment of resistance as a sign or a clue for growth? What if we realize, "Oh, I see what's happening, I'm actually only one step away from being on the plus side of growth; I just don't see it yet."

Now when you look at this graph, you can see that you are on a path to greatness and that this little bit of uphill resistance is actually the world challenging you to become better and grow. You can't grow without friction or resistance, yet we all try to avoid it! However, you can choose to let it ignite you instead!

Growth Mindset

When it comes to losing weight holistically, you also must cultivate a growth mindset while you cultivate your faith. Dr. Carol Dweck talks about this concept in her book *Mindset.* Essentially, Dr. Dweck noticed that the most successful people in life are the ones that purposely develop a growth mindset versus those that have a fixed mindset. A fixed mindset is just like it sounds; you believe change is bad and enjoy it when everything is the same and fits within your bubble. A fixed mindset is a belief that your qualities are carved in stone. You only have a certain amount of intelligence, a certain personality, a certain moral character, etc. People with fixed mindsets don't want feedback because they believe the feedback is a negative knock on their very being.

Conversely, a growth mindset is based on the belief that your basic qualities are things you can cultivate through your efforts. Everyone can change and grow through application and experience. People that have growth mindsets can also take constructive feedback and use it to improve.

In my past life as a police officer, I witnessed the negative power of the fixed mindset and the positive power of the growth mindset. At one point in my career, I was lucky enough to be part of the training division. I would actively train officers just starting their career in the Academy, and I would train veteran officers. I specifically remember training a group of high-level officers and running them through simulation drills where the officers are placed in realistic scenarios and then forced to react using what are, essentially, paintball bullets. It's the most realistic type of training an officer can experience other than real-life scenarios.

We ran two different groups of officers through this training, and both groups failed to some extent. After each scenario, we would give the group feedback so they could learn lessons from the drill and then use that feedback to perform better in the field. One group of officers was noticeably resistant to receiving the feedback and made comments such as, "Yeah, well I don't think we'd ever be put in a scenario like that, so that's why I did what I did." Instead of absorbing the lessons from the drill, these officers were taking personal offense to any critique of their failures and were making excuses and deflecting. The second group of officers experienced the same failures and got the same feedback. But, their reaction was drastically different. There was a ton of open communication and dialogue amongst the group about what went well and what didn't. The feedback was exactly the same. The only difference was what one group decided to do with that feedback moving forward. I walked away from that incident noticing just how powerful both mindsets are, but how much better it is to embrace the power of a growth mindset.

Life Is an Experiment

From this and other experiences, I learned that life is so much more fulfilling, enjoyable and positive if we can actively remove ourselves from our negative emotions. In other words, we can be more scientific in our approach to our own problems and efforts and, in doing so, be more fruitful in our accomplishments. By treating our attempts to do something new as an experiment, we interpret our problems with fewer emotional burdens. When you realize it's just an experiment and you tried something that didn't work, now you can try something new and see if it works. You become a scientist in a lab, looking for new ways and new possibilities to achieve your desired results. It becomes fun and exciting instead of disappointing and heartbreaking when your experiment fails.

This was confirmed for me when I interviewed James Altucher, best-selling author of *Skip The Line,* a book that highlights how to reach your goals and succeed in life without spending 10,000 hours on one subject to develop mastery. What James discovered is that, to get to your goals much faster, you need to run 10,000 mini-experiments rather than devoting 10,000 hours to mastering any skill, habit, goal, etc. Each time you run an experiment, you get some immediate feedback. Take that feedback, reiterate, and run another experiment. Continue to do this until you finally hit your goal. So, instead of thinking that you failed in life, what if you thought, "I just ran an experiment, I got some feedback, and now I can improve and try to run a new experiment based on what I learned from the first experiment?" You never really fail. You're just constantly learning and getting feedback from life. If something doesn't work, good. Now, you know you need to do something different. Test, retest, and repeat.

James not only writes about this, he also embodies this principle to the fullest. This is why he's a chess master, serial entrepreneur, angel investor, best-selling author, has a number-one ranked podcast, and started over 20 businesses - 17 of which failed. He makes it a daily practice to write out multiple new ideas although he knows that nine out of ten of the ideas are complete garbage. But he also knows that one is probably worth paying attention to. The ideas he thinks are worth devoting energy to, he quickly tests them as we mentioned above, gets immediate feedback, and the idea either does well or it flops. But, he doesn't waste years sitting on the sidelines waiting for the perfect time or making sure everything is perfect to execute this one idea. He tests it immediately.

I've used this principle successfully with all of my coaching clients. When I meet with a client one-on-one in our weekly check-ins, and they tell me, "Ah man, I slipped up; I had a bad week." My response is always, "Great! We got some good feedback." They usually look at me, puzzled. I tell them, "Listen, thank God this happened early on while you were in the coaching program with me and not when the program is over." Because that's real life, setbacks happen. But they aren't the end. They are just a new beginning. They initiate the process of zooming out and asking ourselves, "Why didn't that work? Why did I eat horribly this week? Why didn't I hit my workouts this week?"

The usual response clients will tell me is," Oh man, I was so busy this week, I had to work extra hours; I don't know what happened." But when we look closer, we see they weren't doing their daily mindset work so they weren't priming their brain or their reticular activating system (which we'll talk more about later in the book) to direct any focus towards their weight loss goal. Due to the fact that they were working so much, they didn't have time to prep healthy meals in advance and were victims to fast food or whatever food was available and convenient. Lastly, they failed to get in any workouts for the week because their priorities were unclear. Because their mindset work was shoddy, their focus was on how busy they were instead of asking themselves, "What's actually possible?" I don't care how busy you are; most people have ten minutes a day to do some type of movement practice or workout. Instead, they let the belief in their brain that ten minutes won't do any good lead them to think "so why do it at all?"

But, notice here how much good information and feedback we can get from running this scenario as a quick experiment? Let's say that Client A tried to stick to their new healthy lifestyle, but due to the excessive amount of hours put in at their job, they were unable to hit their goals. This is honestly nothing new and has been the story of their lives. They tell all their friends, "I'm just so busy, I have no time." They probably even wear it as a badge of honor. Unfortunately, the idea is sabotaging them from reaching their health goals. So for this client, I might say, "Let's just experiment by doing our daily mindset work again this week and nothing else, and see if that makes a difference in your eating habits throughout the week. If it does, then we got some positive feedback, and let's keep doing more of that! If it doesn't, great, let's experiment some more. Let's try adding daily mindset practice and making sure we have the bare necessities in our fridge to meal prep or some healthy snack alternatives stocked regularly, so we aren't the victims of fast food." Then we can follow up by asking, "Did it work or not?" No matter what, continue to experiment and have fun.

Limiting Beliefs

You will find that many of the truths we cling to depend greatly on our own point of view.

-Obi Wan Kenobi

However, after working with many clients, I've noticed that people can suffer from deep-seated beliefs that limit their ability to approach their health and weight loss journey from this more detached, experiment-oriented, fun point-of-view. Instead, they are hampered by limiting beliefs that seem to have been embedded in their subconscious at an early age. I know this has been true even for my own health and wellness journey.

This is a result of normal human development – which is both bad news and good news. First, the bad news: this affects all of us and stems from developmental processes that were beyond our control because they happened when we were young. Experts in child development will tell you that a child's personality is essentially solidified from the ages of 0-7 years old. It has been explained to me that the brain is in a developmental state during those years where it absorbs all the information around it like a sponge and tries to make sense of life. After the age of seven, the child's brain changes states and continues to develop, but the information absorbed into the brain during those 0-7 years will play an extremely critical role in the person's development for the rest of their life.

This is why clients in their 30's and 40's will often still walk around with old beliefs such as, "I'm not good enough," or "my voice doesn't matter," or "I'm overweight because my family was overweight." When I start to peel the onion and dive into these beliefs and where they come from, it's no surprise that clients can recall a time as a young child when a specific incident or altercation caused them to develop this belief. Because these beliefs are embedded in our subconscious for so long ago, it's hard for people to realize they're even acting out these beliefs as an adult until someone like me, a loved one, or another practitioner brings awareness to the issue.

I know this to be true from personal experience because I still struggle with this old belief that "I'm not good enough." The only thing I can recall from when I was a child in the 0-7 time frame that could account for this struggle was this one instance when I returned home from school with a spelling test. The rule in my house was that I had to give all my tests to my mother and show her my results. I handed my mom the result of one of my spelling tests. I had received a 95%. My mom looked at it and replied, "Good Joel, but how come you didn't get 100?" At that moment, I remember feeling like a huge failure. I felt like, "If I don't get good grades or get a 100%, my mom won't love me as much."

Logically, I know that's not true. My mom loved me very much and wanted to push me toward excellence. My mom was probably genuinely curious why I hadn't gotten a perfect score. After all, we had studied the night before, and I got 100% then. However, my developing brain seems to have interpreted that moment as "I'm not good enough." So, to this day, I have to work at reprogramming these old limiting beliefs because that idea of "I'm not good enough" consistently will reappear in my business, my marriage, my parenting, and much more.

Now for the good news. Luckily, with knowledge comes power. When we understand this about ourselves, we can take steps to exert control over minds and reprogram these old, limiting beliefs. I'm going to show you how throughout this book.

Beliefs and Weight Loss

The evidence shows that we inherit and transmit behaviors, emotions, beliefs, and religions not through rational choice but contagion.

-Dr. Marsden

Let me share with you a powerful story about the enormous influence that our beliefs have over our ability to get healthier and lose weight. A famous study was once conducted on hotel maids, and it was reported in *Psychological Science.* The researchers noted that, just by being "told that the work they do (cleaning hotel rooms) is good exercise and satisfies the Surgeon General's recommendations for an active lifestyle," the women "perceived themselves to be getting significantly more exercise than before," and "showed a decrease in weight, blood pressure, body fat, waist-to-hip ratio, and body mass index," compared to those who weren't told this. How crazy is that? They didn't change anything regarding exercise or even implement a new diet plan. All they did was change their beliefs about their same daily activities.

So let me ask you, what do you believe to be true about yourself and your health? How do you define physical health? How do you define healthy eating? Do you believe you're genetically inclined toward obesity or other health issues? Do you believe you'll live as long as or longer than your parents? Do you believe you're aging well or poorly?

Many times with clients, I am amazed to hear the beliefs they have of themselves. They'll tell me things like, "Yeah, well, my parents had diabetes, so it makes sense that I'll probably get diabetes." What!? Type 2 diabetes is usually what they're referring to, and we know this is a lifestyle disease and can be corrected. If you are reading this right now and thinking that you see yourself in this example, please know that I don't say this to shame any of you. Instead, I feel that so many of us have fallen victim to the Western model of disease and medicine where you're overmedicated. Instead of getting to the root cause of any disease or issue, doctors simply throw NSAIDS, anti-bacterials, and other harsh medicines at you. As a result, we see our health through this illness/pharmaceutical loop because we weren't armed with the right knowledge.

There are other common limiting beliefs that affect many of us in our society. For example, one of my clients, let's call her Susie, expressed the very common limiting belief, "Everyone depends on me. I have to support everyone." Before I met Susie, both her parents had died recently, and she had been the caretaker for both of them. She also was an ex-bodybuilder and a gym owner so she understood diet and nutrition very well and had even helped others achieve their desired physiques. But, when Susie found herself always taking care of everyone else, she never made time for her self-care and actually felt guilty if she took care of herself before she took care of others.

When I asked her where this belief stemmed from, as it clearly wasn't serving her, she told me she could recall an incident when she was five. She was the youngest kid and had three older brothers. One night at the dinner table, there weren't enough chairs for everyone to sit at the table, and the brothers were arguing about who was going to sit at the table. Susie grew sick of all the fighting and bickering and said, "Stop fighting; I'll sit under the table." The fighting stopped, and harmony resumed in the house. But from an early age, Susie developed a belief that she didn't really matter and that she needed to put her own needs on hold for the greater good of others. Do you see how these limiting beliefs can follow us from childhood and wreak havoc on our adult lives if we're unaware of them?

Our ideas about money offer another example of a limiting belief that relates to so many of us. I love asking my clients, "Do you deserve to be wealthy?" Of course, they naturally say, "Sure, absolutely." No, really, think about it for a moment and don't just answer right away: do you *deserve* to be wealthy? If you think the answer is yes, then why aren't you? Many of you might be wealthy, I have no idea. This, of course, also depends on your definition of wealth. But let's just assume I'm talking about a large enough amount of money that would make you feel so secure that you could buy whatever you want and never even have to worry about money. As a matter of fact, you could work whenever you felt like it because even if you missed a day or two of work, you don't NEED the money.

What's fascinating is that many people will come up with all these reasons and justify why they're not wealthy and that it's not a big deal for them to be wealthy. Ask yourself, do you worry about money, or do you have to budget and worry about how much you spend? Most of you would say, "Yes." So at the end of the day, there's a feeling of lack regarding money. There's a feeling of scarcity. Now ask yourself how many of these feelings come from childhood beliefs we learned as kids. Our parents told us things like, "Hey, make sure you eat all the food. We don't waste stuff. This costs *money."* Or what about, "Hey, what do you think, money just grows on trees?" The residual affect is intensified for those of you who came from single-parent homes or homes where your parents struggled to make money. Those same concepts and ideas then manifest in our adult life. We embody this idea of scarcity and lack of finances and money, and we don't even know why. We're simply running on auto-pilot, playing the program we learned from our parents.

The same thing comes up for weight loss, particularly in terms of limiting beliefs about healthy foods. I hear all the time that healthy eating is hard – that healthy food tastes disgusting. That's a belief. But, what if you believed that healthy eating could be nutritious and yummy?

Here's the deal, your subconscious mind does not argue with you. It accepts what your conscious mind decrees. If you say, "I can't afford it," your subconscious mind works to make it true. Select a better thought. Instead, say, "I'll buy it because, in reality, I can afford it. I accept it in my mind."

ACTION STEPS

1. **Examine Your Daily Life:** Look at your life and all the things you do on a daily routine on auto-pilot. Evaluate your day and ask yourself if there's any part of your day you question why you do what you do. Why do you have an 8-5 job, for example? Is that because you have to,

and that's just how life is given your circumstances? Or is it because no one challenged your belief that an 8-5 job is not the only way to make money? Look at your relationships and your marriage. Why are you with this person? Or why do you constantly choose the wrong person in relationships and get heartbroken? Look at your diet and your relationship with food. Do you eat six meals a day because someone instilled the belief in you that it's good for your metabolism?

2. **Prune Your Beliefs:** Look at any of the beliefs that don't serve you and help you reach your higher self and support your vision or your mission. Get rid of that belief and form a new one that supports you. Write it down in a journal, and review it in the morning and at night before you go to bed to help prime your mind and rewire your subconscious so you can start living into a new belief.

3. **Do the Ideal Day Exercise:** Go through your day and imagine what your life would be like if you lived your most perfect, ideal day. Start with the morning, and, almost minute by minute, ask yourself what you'd be doing. Would you be doing the same job you'd be doing? Would you wake up early or late? Whom would you be with? Where would you be living? Then move your way to lunch and then to dinner. Minute by minute, note the things you'd be doing on this ideal day. What would the most perfect day look like? Compare that to your current reality, and ask yourself why there's such a gap between the two. Start making changes to get closer to living that Ideal Day.

Blame/Responsibility

Any time I start coaching a new client with weight loss issues, I'm always curious about what's holding them back and why they're not getting the results they deeply want to achieve. Whatever their individual story is, I do see that all my clients are making one common error. They are breaking the law of the E + R = O equation. This equation is:

$$E \text{ (Event)} + R \text{ (Response)} = O \text{ (Outcome)}$$

I learned this equation many years ago from author, speaker, and high performance coach, Jack Canfield, and watched how it related to my life. Many times we see our results, our (O) Outcomes, and blame them on the external forces in our lives. For example, if someone cuts you off in traffic (the (E) Event), we often blame that person and start cursing and muttering to ourselves. Maybe we even speed up to catch them to follow close behind them (the (R) Response). This leads to road rage, anger, a less vibrant state, maybe an accident, and maybe even, at some point, a physical altercation (the (O) Outcome). Later, we'll justify our (R) Response and say, "Oh well, it wasn't my fault. That asshole cut me off, and I had to…" Even if you don't go as far as following the person and trying to get revenge and you just become irate in the car, you're still letting that person cause you to become angry. You're letting that person take away your happiness, joy, and vibrant state. You're letting that person take away the time from you that you want to devote to becoming your higher self and truly carrying on the higher mission you set forth in life. Why? Why let them steal that from you?

This is even worse if you are a parent with your kids in the car. I lived and worked in San Francisco for many years and encountered some of the most world-class, incompetent drivers. Knowing this, I worked hard to control my (R) Response to (E) Events on the road when my son was in the car. When someone cut me off, I'd laugh and mutter, "Wow, what a moron." That's a much better response than getting extremely angry and looking for revenge, but my son would hear me and ask, "Dad, what happened? Why'd you say that? Who's a moron?" My son would hear me and repeat everything I muttered out loud. Even though I didn't think I was reacting badly, my reactions were having a cause-and-effect relationship with my son. My (R) Response to the (E) Event caused an undesirable (O) Outcome. My son felt the need to stick up for me, and I caused him to be stressed for no reason just because I didn't choose an appropriate (R) Response.

The ironic thing is that the (E) Event part of the equation will always be the same – it will always be something that we can never change no matter how badly we want to try and control it. Trying to control it is where our resistance to change and discomfort arises. Instead, we need to come to terms with accepting that the (E) Event is something that "just is." There's nothing for us to change. There's nothing for us to try other than to "just be," and then life becomes so much simpler.

From that space, we can respond accordingly. This is where we have control. We always have a choice in our (R) Response even when we don't feel like we do. In a completely different context, I remember one of my mentors, self-defense expert Tony Blauer, calling this a "choiceless choice." Tony stated once at a seminar, "When your life is possibly in danger, you have no choice but to fight back. It's a choiceless choice to make. You know in life, you will be met with resistance, so make the choice to accept it and move forward."

The world might have wronged you and dealt you a shitty hand. It might even be unfair, and you don't deserve it (the (E) Event). But at the end of the day, you still have a choice: What will be the (R) response that will help to alter the (O) Outcome?

To grow, you need to decide to stop complaining and to stop spending time with complainers and get on with creating the life of your dreams.

ACTION STEPS

1. **Apply E + R = O:** Evaluate your own life and plug this formula into your life. How often do you blame others and complain about the outcomes in your life? Do you take full responsibility for where you currently are in your life?

2. **Practice Your R's:** Think of an example in your daily or weekly life where you don't take full responsibility in your life or where your response could be a lot better to help

create a more fulfilling or positive outcome. What small thing could you implement right now, today, or this week to help positively shift that outcome?

3. **Stop Complaining:** Best-selling author Tim Ferriss ran an experiment where the rule was that he was not allowed to complain for 21 days. If he did, then he had to start the 21days all over again. He wore a little bracelet on his wrist to remind him. Try going a day without complaining. It's pretty hard. Make it a game and include your friends. Make a wager that the first one to complain has to buy dinner or something else fun. Imagine what your life would be like without complaining. You'll start to notice how triggered and wired we are to complain about everything and look for the bad. But you will also notice that the more you look for the good, the more good you'll find.

Forgiveness Can Get You to Your Goals Quicker

"Wait, what? This guy is talking about forgiveness now? You've got to be kidding me. When are we finally going to get to the losing weight part?" Fear not. I promise we will get there.

In fact, we are there! I can assure you that forgiveness and weight loss go hand-in-hand. After coaching hundreds of individuals, I started seeing a recurring pattern. People's past, their beliefs, and even some of their hardships continue to hold them back in their present life until they've properly dealt with these issues. When your energy is off, your vibration is off, your connection with the world is off, you will just go on accomplishing less, impacting people less, and never reaching your fullest potential.

So, how do we know that forgiveness will help you to gain control over those past issues and thereby enable you to better achieve your goals in your present life? Science, tradition, and experience all show that forgiveness can actually help you manifest or reach your goals faster.

In Vishen Lakhianis' new book, *The Six Phase Meditation Method*, he talks about attending a brain health institute that utilizes advanced neurofeedback to intensively reprogram the brain and help unlock one's potential. He learned from the scientist there that forgiveness not only increases your peace of mind, it actually increases your brain's alpha wave levels (the part of your brain activity that helps you to feel calmer, more creative, and better able to learn new information). Forgiveness, then, is like magic. It can change your world in the blink of an eye. Or, as the scientist explained to Lakhiani, people who practice forgiveness just seem to get "luckier." Your desires and your dreams come true faster and more easily.

Traditional Eastern medicine similarly shows the link between emotions and how your body functions physically. In fact, in Eastern medicine, certain organs are associated with certain emotions. For example, anger is often associated with the liver. If you're someone who is frustrated, angry, stressed, and regretful and stuck in these negative emotions, you also might have issues with what is called 'Qi stagnation' in the liver. You might experience issues such as cold hands, tinnitus, headaches, neck pain, and pain that moves around the body. When we think about optimum health, I'm looking at the whole body as a system and seeing what might need to be tweaked to achieve optimum performance. Emotions, mindset, and beliefs all play a critical role in your health so letting go of negative emotions, mindsets and beliefs is imperative.

My experience with my clients has only strengthened my belief in this mind-body connection. I will ask them, "Think about someone who has hurt you. Is there anyone you just haven't forgiven? Is there a situation you just cannot get past?" Many times we've been hurt by a relative or family member in the past, and I've heard people tell me, "Joel, I just can't forgive that person. Sorry, I won't…" I can relate to that, and I understand that raw emotion. It's painful. It's easy for someone like me to say, "Forgive that person. It'll make you feel better." Or, "You know, in Chinese medicine, they say…"

However, I also recognize that, in theory, we all know what we should be doing, but putting it into practice can be just too painful. With this in mind, I know that many of you will have difficulty letting go and forgiving someone who has hurt you. I understand that. So, at the end of the day, if your pain is too great, I suggest that you don't need to forgive them yet, but you should try to have compassion for them. The people that have hurt you have been hurt by others, and now they continue to spread their hurt. Send them love. Send them love because they never picked up a book like this before to work on their mindset, beliefs, and well-being. Send them love because no one ever taught them the necessary skills to handle difficult situations. Send them love because maybe they didn't learn those skills, and their ego prevented them from doing the right thing. This an excellent way to release those emotions and feelings that could possibly be lingering in the background and stymieing your path to greatness.

Also, for some of us, we need to understand that it's our own ego holding on to control of the situation. You're holding on because, in reality, you want to feel this pain. You want to hold on to it. It sounds contradictory, but it's true. What are you holding on to this pain for? Most of the time, the person that hurt you either has no idea or has completely moved on in their life and is oblivious to your pain. They could care less, yet you continue to carry it on for them. And it's only hurting you and your health, energy, and vibrant force. The moment you accept life as it is or the situation that hurt you as an event that happened, it loses all its power. It loses all its energy and no longer has a hold of you. In turn, you become more powerful, and you can go on to achieve your goals.

ACTION STEPS

1. **Journal Your Pain:** Grab a journal and write freely about an incident or someone who hurt you, and you need to forgive. Let the pen do all the writing, and don't overthink it. Just let the emotions come out and onto the paper. Once you're done, say "Thank you" to that person and close the book. You can throw those journal pages away if need be.

2. **Do the Compassion Exercise:** Sit quietly with your eyes closed and think of the person who wronged you. You don't need to think about it for too long. It could be done as quickly as two minutes. Imagine sending that person love and compassion. Smile and continue to send them compassion since they need it more than anything.

Gratitude/Abundance

Here we go again! What do gratitude and abundance have to do with weight loss? How about EVERYTHING! When you're on a quest to do more, be more, and give more, the world can tend to knock you down or backward. For many, the journey of weight loss can feel lonely. There are times that you don't even know if what you're doing is working. Sometimes you feel lost. Sometimes you feel like throwing in the towel. So many times I have heard things like, "But Joel, this is ridiculous, I see how my sister eats, and she never gains weight. How is it that I can't lose a damn pound?" We start to judge ourselves. We compare ourselves to others.

We forget why we began this journey. We become filled with doubt. We lose trust and confidence in ourselves. Gratitude breaks all that negativity.

How? Well, gratitude does two things. First, gratitude gives you perspective. Second, gratitude makes you realize the abundance around you.

With the perspective born from gratitude, you will realize and accept that there will be struggles along the way and that part of the struggle is trusting the process and continuing to move forward. Also with this perspective, you will look for the good, look for the small wins, look for the small bits of growth and change even when it might seem infinitesimal. This idea, this mindset, goes far beyond little hacks to change your mindset and reframe your focus. Believe me, these are all useful, and I use them to help re-center myself. But, on a higher level, it's your vibration that's connected to the universe that becomes even more powerful because you can't hold on to anger and fear when you approach life through the lens of gratitude.

Seeing life from this perspective also shifts your thinking to an abundance mindset. You realize that doing things like reading this book in the hopes of improving your body means that you are lucky – there are people who can't even move their limbs, but you get to move freely! You have an amazing body! You have the option to actually work out! Think how lucky you are!

There's a phrase I learned from a parenting expert who frequently says, "When you focus on the good in your child, the good gets better." Anybody with kids knows that they can be disruptive and act out, and sometimes you think to yourself, "God! This little kid is such a punk; he won't behave right ever." You start to think that your kid purposely goes out of their way to be disruptive. But if you change your lens and focus on the good in them, you will see that they are good kiddos doing their best. It changes the entire dynamics of parenting, and you start to see all the amazing things they do, and how rich their minds are, and how sweet they really are. It's the same for you and weight loss.

Now, here's where you might think I'm getting really woo-woo. But I've seen tremendous growth in my own life and my clients' lives when this shift is made. When you start connecting with the universe in a way of abundance, you start to pull the right kind of people and resources into your life. When you start to see that you are enough and there this is enough around you, you stop living in a place of lack and scarcity. You stop acting in desperation mode. You become lighter and more blissful. Even in times of uncertainty, you break through those sticking points because you realize that nothing's impossible. There's nothing to fear, and you have the resources and the ability to get through even the most challenging times.

ACTION STEPS

1. **Start a Gratitude Journal:** Each morning, I like to write down 1-3 things that make me feel grateful. It becomes challenging over time because you feel like you're listing

the same things repeatedly. That's okay because this list does not need to be complicated. Look for simple things to list such as the cup of coffee in the morning and how it lights you up, the house you live in since some people don't even have shelter and sleep outside in the cold, etc.

2. **Take a Breath:** Any time you run into a major problem, and you feel overwhelmed and confused, consider doing this: Stop, close your eyes and take several breaths. Start breathing from your heart by imagining that your heart is doing the breathing. After taking several breaths from the heart, think about that problem of yours. But think about it without going back up to your head. Instead, stay in your heart, your grateful heart, and continue to breathe. What does your heart say? Because the heart knows the answer. The head is great for strategy, but the heart knows the answer. Continue to breathe through the heart and wait for the answer. When you're ready, open your eyes and notice the shift in energy and clarity.

Be Uncomfortable

Along with studying and contemplating the many facets of cultivating the proper mindset, I also started wondering, "What separates someone good from someone great?" In pondering this question, I came to the conclusion that people who achieve greatness are people who are OBSESSED. They are obsessed to the point where being uncomfortable and being put in difficult situations actually invigorates them. I am talking about the kind of people who are similar to the people doing cold plunges. The cold is insanely uncomfortable, but the effects felt afterward are extremely beneficial for neuronal growth, hormones, energy, and weight loss. It even occurred to me that people who are great and achieve the impossible are not balanced. In fact, they are imbalanced. There are parts of their lives where all they do is go deep into whatever study or field they are trying to master, and they spend hours and hours there. Sometimes to be great, you need to be a bit imbalanced. And you need to be uncomfortable.

But being uncomfortable is HARD. It is easy to think that most people just won't put in the hard work – they won't wake up when their alarm clock goes off and they hit the snooze button instead, they say they're tired after work, so they won't go to the gym, and so on. It seems like they just don't want greatness badly enough. This is true to an extent. But is also true that the brain likes to be in homeostasis and hates change. It likes being balanced. It likes being comfortable. It's trying to keep you alive so that you survive and live a long time.

The problem is that on the other side of suffering is greatness. Suffering is actually okay sometimes. When I interviewed Dr. Anna Lembke, bestselling author of the book *Dopamine Nation,* she told me, "the antidote to pain is pain…discomfort can trigger our body's own healing mechanisms." Similarly, David Goggins, the retired Navy Seal, ultramarathon runner, and a generally insane individual who does some of the masochist workouts in the world, has said that, through suffering and putting his body through intense, excruciating workouts, he has learned a concept known as the 40% rule. This means that most of the time, when you think you've reached failure, and you think you've given it everything you got, in reality, you've got an extra 40% to give. Isn't that amazing? The mind places governors on us to prevent us from getting hurt. What if you take the governors off? What are you truly capable of when there's nothing to stop you?

Your mind is so powerful. It can convince you and even help justify that it's ok to rest. It's ok to hit snooze because you need more sleep. It's ok to not workout because you had a tough day. It's ok to have that snack because you deserve it since you've been eating well for most of the day. Instead, when these thoughts come about, you need to realize a couple of things: (1) smile and say to your mind, "thank you for being here, I see you, thank you for protecting me" (2) detach for a moment, zoom out and look at what's happening from afar like you're watching a movie between you and your mind (3) once you've got some space and you can see clearly what's happening, connect with your WHY. (4) Now shift.

When you consciously choose to make that mental shift, you can objectively evaluate your road to greatness in your weight loss journey. Why are you doing this again? Why are you losing weight in the first place? Think of all the pain and suffering and emotional distraught that your weight has caused you. Remember why you started this journey in the first place. You wanted to change. You wanted more for yourself. You wanted to be a better dad/mom or role model for your family. Remember the moments when you look in the mirror and think to yourself, "I look disgusting." Remember the confidence you wanted to feel in your new body, the self-esteem, and self-worth you want to capture in your new body. Most of us are getting lost in the day-to-day transitions, and, because we're not connecting with our WHY, we take shortcuts and slip up. Our why is so much bigger than us. Our why will drive us to unparalleled places. When you don't have a why it's easy to give up. It's easy to snooze in, cheat on your diet, and skip workouts because your purpose is good, not great. When you consistently connect with your why and your purpose, you will find a greater reason to rise to the occasion and do what's necessary to accomplish the goals and the vision you set out to achieve.

ACTION STEPS

1. **Prepare for Greatness:** Look at the ways you're limiting yourself daily. Look at how you let your mind trick you into taking the easy route. Make a plan ahead of time so that when something comes up that might cause you to take the easy route, you have a plan of action set in place that allows you to take the hard route.

2. **Get Comfortable Being Uncomfortable:** Do something uncomfortable every day. Make being uncomfortable the norm. Take a cold shower. Do a hard workout. Do a long fast. Do something that will harden the mind, something that will challenge you daily and push you outside of your comfort zone.

Chapter 2

VIision & Values

I'm looking for a lot of men who have an infinite capacity to not know what can't be done.

-Henry Ford

In the first chapter, I laid down the foundation for what it's going to take to be successful long-term in your weight loss and health journey. Without this solid foundation, I truly feel like you'll take the advice that I'm giving or that of any other fitness guru, and you'll treat it like some crash diet or "get results quickly program." Sure, you might get some great results in the beginning, but without the proper mindset and foundation, in the long run, you'll simply fall back into old habits and old limiting beliefs, and you'll end up where you've always ended up - nowhere. I definitely don't stand for that, and I won't let you stand for that either.

Now that you have that solid foundation, or are at least working on it, you need to have clarity and a clear vision for where you want to go. Without clarity, your mission, your goal, and your vision become unclear. It's like the saying, "where focus flows, energy goes." Most people, though, don't focus long enough on their long-term goals, and that's why they don't succeed. Sure, they might focus on it for a week or even a month, but then it starts to lose its energy and focus, and the next thing you know, you're asking yourself, "What happened?" or "Wait, what's my goal again?" This is something you typically see with those New Year's Resolutions. People set these amazing goals to lose weight and get in the best shape of their life, and it lasts for about a month or so, right? In my twenties, I had a membership to Gold's Gym. I was the type of person who went to the gym six days a week. Every January, I'd get so annoyed because the gym was suddenly packed, and you couldn't get in on certain machines. Then, by February, business would return to normal, and the crowds would dissipate. Without fail, this would happen every year.

Why is that? In my opinion, people were never really intentional with what they wanted to achieve, they didn't establish a clear long-term vision, and they weren't connected with their values. In this chapter, we're going to cover all these concepts as well as how to establish the proper goals for long-term growth.

Clarity

When I started my podcast three years ago, I learned this interesting statistic. It said the average podcast lasts only seven episodes. Why? My belief is that the people starting a new podcast had the expectation that they were going to start a podcast, and it was going to be amazing, and they were going to get a ton of downloads and meet famous people, and then they'd kick back and live off of sponsorships as all the big dogs do in the podcasting world. But guess what? After seven episodes, they looked at their download numbers and saw that they were atrocious. No one cared about their podcast, not even their own friends. It's the truth.

I remember when I started and told myself I wouldn't be that stat. To this end, my first step in launching my podcast was to work on establishing a clear vision for my endeavor. First, I knew very clearly that my goal for starting my podcast was to share knowledge that I felt wasn't well known in the health and wellness world. It was clear to me that I had been blessed in my health and wellness journey and education and that other people's podcasts had changed my life. From this clarity, came my vision for my podcast. I deeply and thoroughly know that my 'why' for my podcast is so deep. Secondly, it was clear to me that my vision for my podcast was that it had to be about sharing and not about profiting. My 'why' for my podcast is not so that I can become rich and famous and kick back on endorsements. In the three years of my podcast, I haven't taken a single sponsorship, and it is only recently that people have reached out to me regarding potential sponsorships. In fact, I've spent well over $30k just producing the podcasts, paying editors to cut up clips, etc., yet I still do it for the pure love of trying to help others in their health, weight loss and life-improving journeys. All the while, I have remained clear in my vision - connecting regularly with experts and people smarter than me so I can share their ideas with the world is one of my favorite things to do in life.

This level of clarity and vision extends well beyond my podcast. The other day my coach (yes, I am a coach with a coach – this is how I know that coaching works!) asked me, "Joel what's your why…?" And I told him, "transformation." It is what ignites my passion. There's nothing greater than seeing a client change in positive ways right before your eyes - watching them lose weight, gain more self-confidence, start a new business, ditch old friends and old beliefs and embrace change, take risks and take bold and courageous action. I live for that transformation. That drives me more than money or anything else. If I was driven by money, I would have given up long ago. Being a CEO or an entrepreneur is not easy. The path of growth is not linear. You don't punch in like a 9-5 job every day and then just check out. The business is always going, and there are a lot of highs but also a lot of lows. Being able to weather the lows is what separates the people who make it and the people that don't. Having a clear vision and clear focus on my 'why' and what my vision is for the world is what prevents me from ever stopping.

So what's your 'why?' What ignites your passion? What drives you more than some external goal, like "I want to look better in photos," or "if I'm healthier, I'll make more money…."

I will wager that if you are reading this book, then your 'why' is not so superficial or limited. When I have intake calls with clients, they tell me some profound stuff and it is very inspiring to hear their 'why's'. They tell me they are committed to losing weight and getting healthy because they want to be there for their kids and leave them a legacy of good health. They want to make their kids proud. They want to be happy again because they know that happiness will radiate to others in the world and that lightness in them will transcend themselves and influence others. They want to be a motivational speaker, or change careers, or be a better leader for the people in their community.

Once you're clear on your 'why' and what you're committed to, you must have a clear vision. In many ways, your 'why' and your vision are very similar. The difference is, can you actually envision yourself achieving your goals and living and breathing your 'why' every single day. Multi-millionaire and serial entrepreneur David Meltzer taught me this and said, "Joel, most people are just getting in their own way of achieving their goals. I just remove the interference so that I can actually reach and attain my goals." Remember what I said about those old, limiting beliefs in chapter one? The minute things start not going your way, and you experience setbacks is the moment you experience interference and blockages. You revert to those limiting beliefs of doubt, fear, and scarcity, and you give up on your goal. This is why it's crucial to be connected to your vision no matter what happens.

Visualization

Visualization is an awesome tool for reprogramming those negative thoughts so you can, instead, move positively in the direction of your goals with both clarity and vision. However, most people don't visualize their goals or dreams happening because they think visualization doesn't work. In fact, I used to feel the same even after all of the self-development books I read and seminars I attended suggested that I practice visualization.

That changed when I came to understand the science behind visualization. Remember, most people's subconscious thoughts are full of fears, lack, and scarcity. This is what's constantly running in the background for most people. Neuroscience suggests that 95% of our decision-making is based on these subconscious thoughts and feelings, and only 5% is based on the logical processing part of the brain. How, then, can you honestly achieve greatness and reach your highest potential with those negative thoughts, feelings, and emotions sabotaging you and, sometimes unknowingly, running in the background?

Well, if we know that 95% of our decision-making and what we do regularly is based on the subconscious, then we can make the wise choice to focus on improving these subconscious thoughts. To start, we can understand that our subconscious thoughts are not necessarily *true* thoughts. A famous study known as the Leahy Study of Cornell University showed that humans think thousands of thoughts per day, with 95% being the same as yesterday and 80% being negative. The study also concluded that 97% of our worries are baseless and result from an unfounded, pessimistic perception.

Moreover, when you consistently visualize, you can reprogram your subconscious. This is possible because you activate the part of your brain known as the reticular activating system (RAS) when you practice visualization. ***The Reticular Activating System*** (RAS) is a bundle of nerves at our brainstem that filters out unnecessary information so the important stuff gets through. Your RAS takes what you focus on and creates a filter for it. It then sifts through the data and presents only the pieces that are important to you. All of this happens without you noticing, of course. The RAS programs itself to work in your favor without you actively doing anything.[1] Pretty awesome, right? When I learned these facts, I started taking my visualization practice much more seriously.

In doing so, I also discovered that there are two reasons that people fail at establishing a truly productive visualization practice. These reasons are: (1) it requires constant repetition (you don't do it enough), (2) you don't do it long or deep enough. Instead, you need to create a deep enough emotional charge around the visualization because emotions are what actually embed memories. The neat thing is our brain doesn't know the difference between something vividly imagined and something that actually happened. Therefore, you can help

---

1   "Reticular formation," Wikipedia, accessed April 3, 2023, https://en.wikipedia.org/wiki/Reticular_formation#Ascending_reticular_activating_system.

reprogram your subconscious and all those negative, limiting, old beliefs by using visualization as your friend.

To do so, I recommend connecting with your vision by writing it down daily. I like to do it in the mornings right after I wake up. Visualize in great detail your mission, your goals, your 'why.' Are you pain-free? Are you free of all diseases? Are you open, relaxed, and in an ecstatic state of bliss all day long? Are you flexible as well as strong? Do you exercise, eat good food and drink lots of water? How much do you weigh?

I can't tell you how much this practice has changed my life over the last two years. When I left my job with the San Francisco Police Department, I thought I would go bankrupt and my family would be homeless. Talk about living in a state of fear and uncertainty, right? Even amongst all these fears, I continued to practice my visualization daily and imagined myself crushing my income goals, making a difference and transforming lives and hitting new plateaus in my business. The more I did this practice, the more serendipitous coincidences would occur. A new email would come in with someone saying they wanted to work with me. I would connect with a new thought leader who would connect me with someone else who could actually help my business grow. The more I connected at a higher frequency and continued to visualize myself accomplishing and reaching my goals, the more amazing things were happening in my life.

So let's use the power of the RAS through daily visualization and start bombarding our subconscious with the positive thoughts and imagery that show us achieving the goal, living our best life, moving without pain, breaking through our addictions, hitting our weight loss goals, connecting with our spouses and kids and laughing and loving, etc.

ACTION STEPS

1. **Establish a Routine:** It is best to set up a time in the morning after you wake up or right before you go to bed for this visualization practice.

2. **Visualize Your Goals:** Spend 15-20 minutes visualizing yourself already having accomplished your goals. I usually have 3-5 big goals at a time, and I imagine myself with the energy and vibrancy created around the goal. I may visualize what it would feel like to hit the stage and speak to thousands. Others may visualize receiving awards, hitting their income goal, hitting their weight loss or physique goal, being pain-free, being an amazing father and having beautiful relationships with your kids and spouse, etc.

3. **Find What Helps You:** I personally like to use music and sometimes breath work while I do these visualizations since having a voice or guide seems to help me. There are several apps out there that help with the visualization process. However, one of my personal favorite tools for guiding my visualization is the BrainTap device. You can check out my podcast interview with Dr. Patrick Porter to learn more about why I'm so bullish on this device. I think it can greatly impact your subconscious. For a discount on the device, use the code JOELEVAN at the checkout.

Values

Clients always tell me, "Joel, I'm just not motivated…I don't have the willpower to stop eating." How often do you feel this way? It's a very common and reoccurring theme I see in the weight loss space, and the fact is that statement is just not true. You don't have a motivation problem or a willpower issue. *This is the WILLPOWER Myth.*

Your real problem is that you have no idea what you stand for. You have no idea what your core values are. Let me explain.

Most of you have yet to sit down and think about your strengths. What do you stand for? Whom do you want to be every day? When people think of you and the type of person you are, what do they say? Do they say, "He's hardworking," or "She's thoughtful and caring," or "He's someone of integrity?" You need to be very clear about what it is you value in life and who you say you want to be. Otherwise, you're just going through life unclear, with no vision, just flying by the seat of your pants, hoping and wishing the next day will be great. Even worse, every day just passes you by, and it's the same. There's no growth. There's nothing that ignites your desire to get out of bed and say, "Yes!"

When you're not clear on your values, you let the day control you. You let other people's emotions burden you. Going back to the metaphor of someone cutting you off in traffic, if someone cuts you off and flips you off, how do you react? Do you let their anger dictate your response, or do you align with your values and pivot? What about when your significant other makes a snide remark, is disappointed in you, or gets into an argument over something petty? Do you let their emotions rob you of your happiness and joy? Or do you pivot and align with your higher self?

So how do your core values relate to weight loss? Well, with me, for example, health is one of my core values. Health is something that I really value because I know that when I take care of my health, I feel better, I have more energy, I'm more vibrant, I know I'll live longer and be there for my kids, and I know I will serve my clients in a higher way. So, when I'm on the road and go to a restaurant or I'm at a kid's birthday party with food that's not organic, made with vegetable oils, is heavily processed, and I know is not going to serve me well, that's when I connect with my values. Before being tempted to eat some unhealthy food, I ask myself, "Whom do I want to be right now? Whom do I say I am?"

So, at such moments, I breathe, and I align with my core value - health. Once I'm aligned with health, then willpower and temptation no longer become an issue. These extraneous things no longer hold power over me. Because I'm so certain and so aligned with who my higher self is, something like processed food no longer becomes a thought. I'm no longer wasting energy trying to *will* myself to not do something. I'm no longer struggling with this emotion. Instead, I just am. I'm just being. I'm connected. I'm grounded. When you're not grounded, that's when you slip up.

You see, most people try to fight and struggle and produce more willpower, and it's just not possible. Let's face it, we all live busy, busy lives. We have kids, a mortgage, and jobs (sometimes multiple). We don't get enough sleep, we're distracted by technology and our phones, and, by the time we're confronted with a choice of what we're going to eat for dinner or lunch, we simply can't make a smart, rational decision. We're so exhausted and overburdened that we fail when we try to tap into more willpower to not eat something. We just can't. But if you take that pause for a second and connect with your higher value of health, or whatever it might be, you become aligned. And when you're aligned, it becomes effortless because you're just being. There's no struggle.

ACTION STEPS

1. **List Your Values:** Take a moment and write down your top one, two or three values. Ask yourself the questions: Whom do I want to be every day? Whom do I say that I am? What's an emotion I want to feel every day? When people are asked what kind of person I am, what do they say about me? What's a value that I don't embody yet, but I want to start embodying?

2. **Commit To Your Values:** This crucial Action Step is simple. Once you figure out what your top values are - commit to them.

3. **Be Prepared:** Have a plan in place for when you might be tempted to eat something that won't serve you

well. Already have it in your mind what you're going to do - if this happens, then do this. There's a lot of neuroscience behind this. Our pre-frontal cortex, the executive decision-making part of our brain, is offline much of the time when we're making these decisions even though we tend to think we're quite logical human beings. But, most of the time, we operate on feelings and emotions and how we're feeling in the moment. We just need to remember that these feelings are transitory. They come and go. If you have a plan in place, your brain will gravitate to that because you've already primed the mind for action. So, instead of being caught-off guard when faced with unhealthy choices, prepare your responses ahead of time. Top-tier military groups apply this principle to their planning. They call it a P.A.C.E Plan: Primary, Alternate, Contingency, Emergency. They have a primary plan based on an incident going 100% perfectly, an alternate plan if it changes, a contingency if the alternate plan fails, and an emergency plan. Applying this way of thinking and preparing to your own life is so important because it takes all of the guesswork out of how you will feel and react when poor food choices come up.

Goal-Setting

As best-selling author and coach Brendon Burchard said, "When you leave your growth to randomness, you'll always live in the land of mediocrity." It's true. Thankfully, there is an antidote to the randomness that results in mediocrity. This is the practice of goal-setting.

Setting goals is common knowledge, and every client I've worked with understands the power of goal-setting. The problem is that very few actually practice it. They say, "Yes, I know I'm supposed to set my goals and write them down." Yet, often when I'm coaching people and ask if they have a journal and write down their goals, they tell me, "No." If you're not tracking where you want to go, how can you measure that what you're doing is working? The purpose of goals is to give you clarity in what you want and what you're trying to attain.

For those clients who do set goals, I've found that most people set goals in the wrong way. It is not enough to think about your goals or to even write down your goals. Not only should you write down your goal, but you want to look at it every day, multiple times a day – at least in the morning and at night. It will not work if you rely solely on your memory about the one time you wrote your goal in your journal. If you wrote "lose weight" in a journal, but never looked at it again or even waited a week to look at it again, then I guarantee your lack of success will reflect that lack of attention. When the brain is not constantly reminded and the subconscious is not programmed regularly, you'll default to your old ways.

Therefore, you must be vigilant and remember that we have a lot of limiting beliefs and past traumas from childhood that make up the majority of our subconscious thoughts. If those subconscious thoughts are not primed for success, your default mindset will take over. You need to constantly be directing and guiding your focus to what's possible for you, whom you need to become, and what you need to do to make what's possible inevitable.

Think of weight loss goal-setting as being like the 'Law of Attraction' which posits that the more good energy you put out there, the more resources, opportunities, and people will come into your life to help you achieve your goals. It seems woo-woo, but I see it all the time. You become a vibrational match for the energy you're putting out in the world so don't let it be pessimistic energy. If you think, "I could never achieve 25 lbs of weight loss in 60 days," then guess what? You won't! You told your subconscious that's it not possible, and your brain will do everything to ensure it doesn't.

On the other hand, amazing things will happen when you take an optimistic approach. In fact, your brain will help you to achieve your goals. When you review your goals multiple times a day, 'structural tension' is created in your brain. Your brain wants to close the gap between your current reality and the vision of your goal. By constantly repeating and visualizing your goal as already achieved, you will be increasing this structural tension. Not only will you create your motivation, but you'll stimulate creativity as your brain seeks new ways to achieve that goal. Moreover, the steps you take to achieve the goal are transformative in their own right. This will always be of far greater value than what you get in the end. In fact, the beauty of goals is that you don't even have to accomplish them, it's about whom you become in the process.

Therefore, you must think globally when you start your goal-setting practice. You need to ask yourself, "What experiences do I want to have in this lifetime? How do I want to grow? How do I want to contribute?" These are the types of questions that are going to expand you and stretch you for the rest of your life. Most of us set goals for things like how much money we want, what college we want to get into, what job we want, etc. Don't get me wrong. Those are all good goals to have at some point in your life. After all, having a successful job that makes you happy and earns you the amount of money you need to survive and regularly provides food and shelter for your family is a good thing. But, after you've accomplished those basic needs, you need to level up your game and look for ways to really expand and stretch yourself.

In terms of weight loss goals, you must give yourself clear *stretch goals.* You need to give yourself deadlines. And you need someone to hold you accountable. That is the fastest way to goal-setting success. You also need to ask yourself what other broader skill sets you will need to master in the coming months and years that will serve you with excellence at the next level. If you're someone who needs to lose 25 lbs in the next 60 days, but you don't know where to start or know how to cut through the noise and eat properly, then what can you do immediately to start changing that? Is it a book you need to read? A coach or trainer you need to hire? Be decisive and take massive action.

ACTION STEPS

1. **Write Down Your Stretch Goal:** Write down something that is not going to be impossible but is a goal that is going to challenge you and make you jump out of your comfort zone.

4. **Review Your Stretch Goal:** Have a journal or a place where you can review this goal at least twice a day. The morning and night are best because that is when your subconscious is most ready and available to take in this information.

5. **Create Accountability:** Share this goal with someone to hold you accountable. There are even certain websites you can join by putting a wager on one of your goals and, if you don't accomplish your goal, the website will automatically donate money to organizations/charities that you don't like!

Scan the QR code below to get a list of resources I use regularly to maintain a sharp mindset.

Chapter 3

Cravings and Habits

"Food-addicted brains are not happy brains."

-Mark Schaztker

The Origin of Cravings

In the last chapter, we explored the damage that can arise from buying into the WILLPOWER myth. You learned that you may actually suffer from a lack of connection to clearly visualized core values versus suffering from a lack of willpower. The reason long-term weight loss tends to fail is the inability of folks to regulate their appetites. Most people trump this up to a willpower issue and fall back on the excuse that they're just not strong enough to resist delectable temptations. Cravings play a huge role in this kind of dysregulated appetite, and I often hear folks say, "I just can't control myself." But, in my research and in my connection with many experts in this field, cravings seem to be more of a brain chemistry problem than a willpower problem. The cool thing about this is that, once you understand what's going on in your brain, you can hack that process and disrupt these cravings for good.

The desire to eat is hardwired into our brains in many ways and involves neurotransmitter pathways. The first neurotransmitter you should understand in relation to cravings is dopamine. Most people think dopamine is a pleasure-seeking neurotransmitter, but that's actually not true. Evidence shows that dopamine is actually all about incentive. Dopamine is motivation. Dopamine is excitement. Dopamine is that get-up and go! Dopamine is desire. But - and this is important to understand - not all desire is dopamine. People desire world peace, but that's not the same type of desire connected to dopamine. Instead, dopamine desire is a powerful "wanting." Dopamine is craving.

The second neurotransmitter pathway that you must understand in relation to cravings is the "liking" pathway. "Liking" is the *enjoyment* of whatever you were "wanting." "Liking" is the impact moment of pleasure. This "liking" is separate from "wanting." "Wanting" is what makes you put a piece of delicious triple-layered chocolate cake in your mouth. "Liking" is what may happen when you taste that cake. It is not a dopamine thing. It has its own brain circuitry with a different set of neurotransmitters that trigger opioid receptors. So, from a neurological perspective, "wanting" and "liking" are different.

In fact, research about binge eating illuminates the critical difference between "liking" and "wanting." Studies show that binge-eaters are struck by thoughts of food even when they aren't hungry. They're filled with overwhelming anticipation, an intense "wanting," for the food. This is a classic sign of dopamine. When researchers showed obese adolescent girls a picture of a chocolate milkshake, they experienced a surge in "wanting." However, these girls experienced a blunted pleasure response when actually drinking chocolate milkshakes. Lots of "wanting," not very much "liking." This is addiction. People suffering from obesity are not gluttonous pleasure-seekers. They are honestly trapped in a cycle of "wanting" – of craving.

How To End Cravings

Anja Hilbert, a professor of behavioral medicine at the University of Leipzig, treats some of Germany's most extreme cases of obesity and disordered eating. Interestingly enough, her experiments showed "liking" can be used as a tool against "wanting." In one of Hilbert's experiments, she explains how she treated a woman who binged on gummy bears. Hilbert gave the woman a Belgian chocolate praline. She asked the woman to close her eyes, put the praline in her mouth, and then let the warmth of her body melt the chocolate and reveal its creamy beauty. Hilbert's patient was instructed to go to the chocolate store anytime she had a huge desire to eat gummy bears, buy just one single praline, and repeat this exercise. Guess what? The woman's desire to eat gummy bears slowly vanished. This dark chocolate "trick" also helped many of Hilbert's other patients with their binge eating disorders. Dark chocolate, which is rich in antioxidants and polyphenols, became a delicious and relatively healthy alternative. By showering the "liking" pathway, the "wanting" pathway was extinguished.

I have adopted this principle in my own life. I love red wine. It is marketed as being "good for you" (in moderation, of course) because it is full of antioxidants. However, staying focused on my core value of health, I decided to do my own research and not trust the marketing. I learned about the toxins, dyes, and chemicals that are put in normal wine. I switched to a biodynamic healthy version like Dry Farm Wines. These wines are practically sugar-free and are tested for mold, glyphosate, and all the other toxins that are disrupting your vitality (if you want to learn more about their wine, check out my interview with Todd White, CEO of Dry Farm Wines, on The Hacked Life Podcast Episode #032).

Yet, even after I had switched to this healthy version, I found that drinking red wine was causing me two issues. First, I noticed myself drinking wine more regularly. It was not excessive, just a glass with dinner every night. But, I did not like that it was becoming a habit. Second, whether I like it or not, wine is alcohol and alcohol is a neurotoxin. And, despite the fact that I was drinking the healthiest wine possible, it started to affect me negatively. I have a sleep tracker and began to notice that my sleep and recovery scores were dropping when I had my glass of wine with dinner.

I realized that I needed to take a break from habitual wine drinking so I researched viable, healthier alternatives. I chose to replace red wine with kava. Kava is a beverage or extract made from the Piper methysticum plant. In the South Pacific, it's a popular drink used in ceremonies for relaxation. Kava can produce some of the same relaxing effects as alcohol, but it does not have any negative side effects. Believe it or not, kava has some interesting properties that can positively effect weight loss by activating a pathway called AMPK (Adenosine Monophosphate Activated Protein Kinase). AMPK activation is responsible for an increase cellular autophagy, a bodily process that involves converting stored body fat and old damaged cells (including cancerous cells) into usable energy as fuel. Check out my podcast with Cameron George, the founder of TruKava, to learn more (Episode #49).

When I stopped drinking wine and started drinking kava instead, I realized how much of a comfort habit red wine had become for me. I also realized that red wine isn't something I need. My "wanting" red wine had skewed my view of its necessity in my life.

As Hilbert learned, "wanting" is stubborn, powerful, and inflexible. No matter how much you try to turn off addictions and use willpower to break that "wanting" cycle, it doesn't work. Dieters and drug addicts know this. However, the two brain circuits talk to each other. They exchange information. By opening the door to enjoyment and showering the body/brain with "liking," we can now get better control over "wanting."

Be Patient With Dopamine

We are hard-wired into wanting immediate results. Luckily, we just learned to be wary of "wanting." So, if you have already decided to try experimenting with something like swapping dark chocolate for a less healthy treat or drinking kava instead of wine, you know to beware of wanting the swap to work like magic. After a week or so, you might ask yourself, "Why am I still addicted to [insert whatever junk food]? It's been a week already." We want immediate results overnight, even though we've been strengthening these dopamine pathways for the majority of our life, and we're hoping for a hack to make it go away overnight. I see this happen repeatedly with clients, and I have to remind them about the process, not the outcome. I want you to always keep things in perspective and remember the long game.

My experience with this was confirmed when I interviewed best-selling author Dr. Anna Lembke. She wrote *Dopamine Nation*, and she told me that, in her clinical experience as well as what is seen in the data, it takes about four weeks to reset dopamine pathways. You'll hear people talk about going on a "dopamine detox" from their phone or whatever addictive habit they try to break. Just understand that resetting those dopamine pathways to a more normal baseline isn't going to be easy. It will take about a month.

But, now that you're empowered with this information, you can smile and relax when only a week has passed and you feel like no real change has happened in your body. The outcome will come, I promise. It just takes time.

ACTION STEPS

1. **Use Your "Liking" Pathway to Curb Your "Wanting" Pathway:** To get better control and prevent food addictions and binge eating, look for positive ways to stimulate the "liking" pathway to dampen the "wanting" pathway. Most people suffering from obesity overindulge; it's the quantity of junk food that's really hurting them. We can prevent that by, instead, indulging in a small quantity of something delicious that we really like. Quality can help combat quantity.

2. **Try the Dark Chocolate "Trick":** Just like in the studies Hilbert conducted, try substituting a healthy piece of dark chocolate for whatever junk food you crave. My personal favorite brand of dark chocolate is <u>Askinosie</u>. I have no affiliation with them, but I appreciate their sourcing and humanitarian efforts. They also make these "itty bitty" bars that are the perfect size for having an after-dinner treat. These will stimulate your "liking" enough to dampen that "wanting" feeling.

3. **Listen to My Cravings-Related Podcasts:** 1. Listen to <u>podcast</u> Episode #152 I did with Mark Schatzker. He wrote the book, *The End of Craving,* where he goes into much more detail about these cravings experiments. I know many of you are wondering how to avoid binge eating salty foods, not just sweets. In this podcast, Mark also tells a great story about how he battled chip addiction. 2. Listen to <u>podcast</u> Episode #55 I did with Dr. Adi Jaffe. He specializes

in addiction and wrote the book *The Abstinence Myth.* 3. Listen to podcast Episode #157 I did with Dr. Anna Lembke. She wrote the book *Dopamine Nation.*

Habits

Cravings and habits are like links in a chain. As my experience with drinking red wine shows, it had simply become a rote habit that was set on autopilot. I didn't even recognize this until I interrupted the habit. Fortunately, as with cravings, habits can be amended when you understand the physiological underpinnings of habits and then use that knowledge to break bad habits and build good habits.

The brain is all about the path of least resistance. You see, the brain likes habits/routines because it limits the number of decisions the brain has to make. Think about how many decisions you have to make daily. Think about how many times you have to be paying attention intentionally. It's a lot of processing and computing power for the brain to always be "ON." This is why the brain looks for shortcuts such as habits. By falling back on habits, the brain conserves energy and its job is made easier. Unfortunately, though, most of us pick up bad habits, especially around eating.

Habit expert, BJ Fogg, explains habit formation in his book *Tiny Habits.* He also talks about using the information about how habits are formed to disrupt bad habits. Understanding how to form a habit is huge when looking at ways to alter or eliminate some of your habits. This is done through recognizing and utilizing the three main drivers of habit formation: Motivation, Ability, and Prompt.

First is Motivation. This driver of habit formation is the most self-explanatory. It is exactly what it says. Motivation is your desire to do or accomplish a behavior.

Second is Ability. This driver of habit formation is more layered. Ability is not just your physical or mental capacity for accomplishing an activity. Ability is also having *access* to this activity. For example, if you were trying to quit drinking, you could remove all the alcohol from your house in order to prevent you from having the Ability to drink.

Third is Prompt. This driver of habit formation is less obvious than Motivation and Ability, yet it is the crux of being able to break bad habits. Prompt is your cue to desire to do the habit. For example, if every night you finish dinner and then sit on the couch, watch TV, and eat junk food, then we could argue that sitting on the couch after dinner is the Prompt that cues your brain to engage in the bad habit of eating junk food. The very act of sitting on the couch after dinner creates a cascade of bad habits such as mindlessly snacking on junk food while watching TV. Conversely, if you remove the Prompt, you can help alter the behavior. So, instead of sitting and watching TV after dinner, walk to another room or go to bed and pick a book to read.

In my own life, I've used the same principles I just outlined to break some bad habits. I also have discussed the effectiveness of these concepts with experts. For example, when I interviewed Dr. T. Dalton Combs, Founder and CEO of Temper, a company that focuses on helping people master their metabolism, he told me that the key to success with the clients in his program is mastering their habits and changing their behaviors. Dr. Combs' program is geared towards fasting and helping people lose weight, yet that's not the secret to his client's success. It's the consistent check-ins and requirements for accountability that help his clients lose the habits that are not serving them well and then cementing new, good habits into their lives.

Forming New Habits

Understanding how a habit is formed is crucial because, once you understand the cyclical mechanisms that cement habits, you can begin to look for ways to break your bad habits. Just as crucially, you can use that knowledge to develop good habits. You take the drivers of Motivation, Ability and Prompt and make them work for you. In developing and maintaining good habits, you convert those drivers. Prompt becomes the Anchor on which to build your good habit. Ability becomes the many Tiny Steps you take in your good habit-building. Motivation becomes the Celebration of your successes along the path to developing and cementing your new, healthy habit.

Let your Prompt become your Anchor. If you're adding a new habit to your routine, look for a way to Anchor it to something you already do. So, for example, let's say it's difficult for you to make working out in the gym a daily a habit. Could you do

20 push-ups a day instead? One of my clients, Cameron, had this very problem. He enjoyed going to the gym, but he was a first responder in a busy city and worked a lot of overtime. He had financial goals he wanted to achieve as well as his fitness goals.

So, we created an Anchor for him to achieve doing 20 push-ups a day. Whenever he came home from work, he entered his home, placed his things down, and did 20 push-ups. This Prompt of entering his house became the Anchor on which he developed his good habit. Entering the house was something he already did regularly, so we knew that Anchoring his new habit to it would stick.

The neat thing for him and many others I've coached is that once you start the habit, it often will lead to more output. The hardest part is getting started, but, once you've started the process, it's much easier to continue. After doing 20 push-ups, you feel so good, and your energy has shifted positively. You'll often end up doing even more push-ups because the momentum has already been created.

Look at your routines and see where you can stack a habit to something you're already doing. There are several habit-stacking techniques, but Anchoring is by far the most effective and the one I've seen that is most effective for anyone looking to form new habits.

Next, be realistic about your Ability and let this guide you in taking Tiny Steps. If you're someone like Cameron who is looking to add a new habit, you should also start small. Think of him replacing an entire workout at the gym with 20 push-ups. Then think of him wanting to do more and more push-ups as his new habit makes him feel better and better.

Now, say you want to develop the habit of going to the gym. You want to operate on one simple premise – take Tiny Steps. Often, when we attempt to create or take on a new habit, we make it big and think we're going to accomplish all this stuff. In reality, we have neglected to take into account our Ability. Then, when we don't accomplish it, we get upset and shame ourselves. So, if you're starting a new habit like going to the gym, make it achievable and break it down into Tiny Steps.

First, drive to the gym, park your car, then leave. Do that for a week or a few days. Once you feel confident with that, drive to the gym, enter the gym, check in, and leave. Your only goal is to go to the gym and then leave. The next time you go, park your car, check in to the gym, lift one dumbbell, then leave. You get the point. You're going to constantly stack on one new piece of the new habit until it becomes a habit. The beauty of this is that you make it so achievable that you can't fail.

But, it seems silly, right? Like, "Joel, really? I'm going to drive to the gym and then leave?" When I interviewed world-renowned fitness coach and supplement formulator Douglas Grant, a top sports nutritionist for many professional teams, I asked him how he got such great results with professional athletes and what he believes to be the key to consistency at such an elite level. He told me, "Easy. It's all about getting small wins and building over time." After 30 years of coaching elite athletes, Doug has built a database of what works and what doesn't work; otherwise, he wouldn't still be in business. He recognizes the importance of getting those small wins and the importance of stacking them over time to create long-term results. Believe it or not, this is the same principle that works with people going to the gym for five minutes and then leaving. At some point, you tell yourself, "Well, I'm already here. I might as well do more."

Pump up your Motivation through Celebration. Another thing to note is that the brain remembers emotions. When working to create and maintain new, healthy habits, you need to keep up your Motivation. You do this by building positive reinforcement through a lot of good emotions. By achieving and celebrating the Tiny Steps as we build a new habit and as we succeed in establishing a new, healthy habit, we're imprinting a positive neuro-feedback loop that makes us want to continue this habit. One of the biggest mistakes with habit formation is not celebrating those wins in order to create an emotional charge that says, "Yes!" Consistently giving the brain this positive reinforcement is highly effective. There are various ways to celebrate, such as moving your body into a power-pose position, listening to a song, or simply making a gesture like Tiger Woods' fist pump.

ACTION STEPS

1. **Break Bad Habits:** Write down a list of all the habits you want to eliminate. Now write down how you can disrupt that habit by attacking either Motivation, Ability, or Prompt. Can you make the habit less desirable? Can you make the habit more difficult to do? Can you change the cue that initiates the habit in the first place?

2. **Develop Good Habits:** Write down a list of all the new habits or a habit you want to start. Follow the model for creating a new habit. Anchor —> Tiny Steps —> Celebrate

3. **Learn More about Habits:** To learn more about habit breaking and habit making, I suggest **that** you read Dr. Fogg's book *Tiny **Habits***.

Scan the QR code below to get a list of resources I use regularly to strengthen my habits and curb cravings.

Chapter 4

Detox

The TSCA (Toxic Substances Control Act) Inventory has continued to grow since then, and now lists more than 86,000 chemicals. (referring to the number of man made chemicals you're exposed to on a yearly basis)

-Environmental Protection Agency's (EPA) Homepage

EMOTIONAL DETOX

Thoughts Are Powerful

You understand that thoughts are powerful. The first three chapters of this book have explored the myriad ways in which your thoughts can shape the struggles and successes in your life – how your thoughts can ignite your passion and your drive, and how your thoughts can ignite the fuel that propels your weight loss journey. It is through thought, belief, and intention that all things happen. Whenever you say or write something down, you're using the energy of your thoughts to affect the world around you.

Now, imagine how your thoughts affect the world *within* you. Everyone has some kind of internal conversation at times. What do you say to yourself? Many people criticize themselves far more often than they praise themselves. I remember attending a parenting seminar, and the instructor said, "You need to be praising your kids with positive reinforcement at a ratio of 8 to 1. Eight positive affirmations for every one negative reinforcement." She assured us that, most of the time, kids are behaving just fine. The real problem is that parents tend to focus more on what their kids are not doing. Remember, "Where your focus goes, energy flows."

Maybe adults need more positive affirmations too – especially in our self-talk – and more focus on the positives that are happening in our lives rather than on the negatives of what isn't happening. Conduct a self-audit of your self-talk and see what you're saying about yourself regularly. You might be completely unaware of your negative self-talk and how much it's hurting you. Or, how often do you complain? Complaining is such a low, negative vibration, and it solves nothing. Instead of complaining, I try to look at things that annoy me or are big problems for me and say, "Thank you." One of my mentors, David Meltzer, taught me this. Saying "thank you" actually reframes life. You begin to see that things are happening *for* you, not *to* you.

When you look at life's challenges this way, you start to welcome and accept the hard things because you know they are going to make you better and wiser and stronger in the end. Also, saying "thank you" is the easiest form of gratitude. And gratitude is the strongest emotion or vibrational frequency that leads to long-term happiness. Even if you don't believe in vibrational frequencies and shifts, you may have experienced the power of intentionally shifting your emotions in a trying situation. Maybe you simply said, "I'm sorry" in a heated argument and that argument fizzled out. Maybe you chose to think, "When one door closes, another door opens," when faced with disappointment, and then the stress of that situation decreased. When my kids are yelling and screaming at each other, I simply say, "Thank you." It sounds ridiculous, but it's changed how I react and engage with them. That alone is worth it. Now those moments will make me a better dad. I know there is a lesson there somewhere, and I'm learning to be more empathetic and compassionate to my kids. Even if I don't see the lesson being taught, I know there is something good there if I look for it.

Experiments have been conducted that show the power of our thoughts and the vibrational shifts that occur when we choose positive thoughts over negative thoughts. In his book, *The Hidden Messages in Water*, Dr. Masura Emoto explains how water exposed to loving, benevolent, and compassionate human intention took on aesthetically pleasing physical molecular formations, whereas water exposed to fearful and harsh human intentions took on disconnected, disfigured, and "unpleasant" physical molecular formations. He did this through Magnetic Resonance Analysis technology and high-speed photographs. Through this pioneering study, Dr. Emoto demonstrated that environment, thoughts, and emotions shape water. Other studies have shown that our thoughts can directly influence the rate of growth in plants, fungi, and bacteria.

Thoughts are Physical

Given the power that our thoughts can have over the external, physical world, we would be silly to think that emotions, thoughts, and feelings don't affect our internal, physical world. Our thoughts definitely affect our health. Any time I've worked with a client, I've always found there to be some type of emotional component behind their illness or weight loss issues. When tracing back your past, ask yourself, "When did weight actually start becoming an issue?" Usually, I'll find some emotional event or a period of difficulty and trauma the client was struggling with that triggered the cascade of poor health and eventual weight gain.

This really hit home for me when I interviewed Dr. Bradley Nelson, author of *The Emotion Code*. He told me that every cancer he ever treated, "had a trapped emotion in the malignant tissue." In *The Emotion* Code, Dr. Nelson explains:

Three things happen when we experience an emotion. First, our body generates the emotional vibration. Second, we begin to feel the emotion and any thoughts or physical sensations that come along with it. Third, we choose to let the emotions go, and we move on after a few seconds to several minutes. This last step is called processing, and once it is completed,

*we have successfully moved on from the emotional experi-
ence, and it shouldn't cause any problems.*[2]

But, as Dr. Nelson further explains, when either the second
or third step is interrupted and the emotional experience is
incomplete, then interference occurs in the body, and the
energy of the emotion is likely to become trapped in the body.
Why are these emotions getting trapped? We don't know
for sure. But, it also seems that the more overwhelming or
extreme an emotion is, the more likely it will become trapped.

When emotions get trapped, you get stuck in the middle of
whatever traumatic event you were experiencing. Instead of
moving beyond your angry moment or a temporary bout with
grief or depression, you retain this negative emotional energy
within your body. This may lead to potentially significant
physical and emotional stress. Believe it or not, trapped
emotions have well-defined energy that has a shape and
form. We can't see them, but they are very real.

Dr. Nelson has countless testimonials from patients he has
treated by helping them to release their trapped emotions.
For example, he had a patient who suffered from chronic pain
for nine years. When he helped that person to release their
trapped emotions, their pain was gone. Another one of his
clients was stuck in the dating world and could never seem to

---

2   Dr. Bradley Nelson, *The Emotion Code: How to Release Your Trapped Emotions
     for Abundant Health, Love, and Happiness* (New York, NY: MacMillan Audio,
     2019).

find the right person. After releasing several trapped emotions, she serendipitously met Mr. Right the following week and has had a thriving, healthy relationship ever since. Dr. Nelson trains practitioners all around the world to do what he does, and the results and testimonies are very much the same.

My own personal and professional experiences have confirmed this link between past emotions and present realities. As a kid, I never had any "real" trauma in the sense of physical or sexual abuse or any outstanding traumatic event that would have left an indelible impression in my mind. However, like any kid, I faced my own demons and micro traumas that I believed were significant at the time, and I can still see when the impact of these issues shows up and affects my adult life to this day. Likewise, whether I'm working with a client on weight loss, detox, gut health, or even something more serious like an autoimmune condition, I have always, and yes, I mean always, found that there was some emotional event that either triggered the condition or was preventing them from getting better. It is really important to note here that this happens although most of my clients never think – or even seem like - they have any *emotional baggage*.

On the flip side, this leads to good news. When my clients have been cleared of their trapped emotions – their emotional toxins – they go through the protocols I recommend for them with greater ease and get faster results.

Bottom line, emotions matter whether you like it or not. More specifically, trapped emotions could be the root cause of many of your struggles. Trapped emotions can interfere with the proper function of your body's organs and tissues, wreaking havoc with your physical health, and causing pain, fatigue, and illness. You need to detoxify your emotional state and shed the weight of your negative and trapped emotions so you can begin the process of successfully shedding some of your physical weight.

ACTION STEPS

1. **Conduct an Emotional Audit:** Think about your emotional responses. Are you super reactive? Are you short all the time with your kids or spouse? Do you overreact to innocent remarks or misinterpret behaviors and find yourself constantly short-circuiting relationships? Even worse, do you suffer from depression, anxiety, and other unwanted feelings that you can't seem to shake?

2. **Journal Your Emotions:** A simple journal exercise consists of: "writing it out to get it out." Journaling helps people put words to emotions with anxiety and loss. Most of us are numb to our emotions. Journaling helps create awareness around those ruminating thoughts. The more we can work through those emotions and identify them, the more space we can create so that we can better cope with anxiety in the future. Dr. James Pennebaker has conducted numerous experiments highlighting the

positive effects of *therapeutic journaling.* The expressive writing protocol consists of asking someone to write about a stressful, traumatic or emotional experience for three to five sessions, over four consecutive days, for 15-20 minutes per session.

3. **Sticky Note** - Write your deepest fear on a sticky note, "I'm boring," "I'm a fraud," or "I'm unlovable." Then stick it on your chest proudly and go introduce yourself to someone. Pretend you're at a party and they put on music. What a relief to see a thought as a thought

4. **Say "Thank You":** Next time you are in a situation where negative feelings are arising, try saying "Thank You" and look at the situation from a more positive perspective. Is there something you can learn from the experience? Did you handle it better than the last time you were in a similar situation and now you know that you are growing as a person?

5. **Seek Professional Help:** Some of you might need to do some deeper work. Connect with a professional therapist, or maybe work with an Emotion Code Practitioner or Life Coach.

PHYSICAL DETOX

It is not a coincidence that the liver is associated with negative emotions. As noted in Chapter 1, traditional Eastern medicine associates the liver with negative emotions such as anger.

This has long been true in Western culture as well and is evident in the English language. "Liverish" and "bilious" are adjectives used for describing irritable, angry people.

Like emotional toxins, chemical/biological toxins pile up in our lives, clutter up our systems and weigh us down from the inside out. These physical toxins get trapped in our bodies and hamper people, including my clients, from reaching their true potential. Like their emotional counterparts, these chemical/biological toxins need to be released from our bodies so we can start making positive changes in our lives.

The Liver, Gallbladder and Bile

Every six minutes, all the blood in your body is circulated through your liver. It is the filter of your blood. The liver removes toxins from your blood and processes them into waste. We need that waste to be properly eliminated from our bodies in order for us to stay healthy.

Our liver detoxes these toxins in two separate phases or 'pathways.'

Phase 1

In the phase 1 pathway, the liver takes a toxin and turns it into a non-toxin by using another compound or mineral in the body to transform the toxin into something that is "waste friendly." You can actually see the end result of this process when you take too much of certain vitamins or mineral supplements and your body ends up excreting the excess quantities in your urine.

More precisely, during phase 1 of the liver's detoxing process, your liver is taking fat-soluble metabolites (toxins) out of your blood and converting them into an intermediary metabolite. This happens by using certain vitamins, minerals, and nutrients like B vitamins, vitamin C, vitamin E, and others.

If you're taking a high-quality, activated multi-vitamin or eating a high-quality and varied diet, you are most likely getting these nutrients daily. For most people, when the liver is provided with quality nutrition, this phase of detoxification is easier for our liver to handle.

Phase 2

But, if your body cannot find a way to turn a toxin into something that is "waste friendly" in the phase 1 pathway, then it passes that toxin off to the phase 2 pathway where the body tries again to convert the toxin. If the phase 2 pathway cannot process the toxin then the body stores it somewhere, such as in adipose (fat) tissue. The key thing to note here is that your body has to have the right nutrients, minerals, and vitamins to turn on both pathways. If it doesn't, those toxins will get stored in the fat tissue.

More specifically, phase 2 is when sulfur-based nutrients like n-acetyl cysteine (NAC), glutathione, and other nutrients such as glutamine and glycine are needed to change the intermediary metabolite into a harmless water-soluble molecule that can be safely excreted through your urine, stool, or sweat.

Phase 2 is typically where I see issues with a client's ability to break down these intermediary metabolites into water-soluble waste. The liver simply lacks the raw material it needs to complete the process at the same rate as the demand placed upon it. When someone lacks these phase 2 nutrients (which are not common in multi-vitamins or the standard diet), they cannot fully remove the toxins. This means your liver then recirculates these toxins back into the blood where they can cause damage and increase your bodily toxic load.

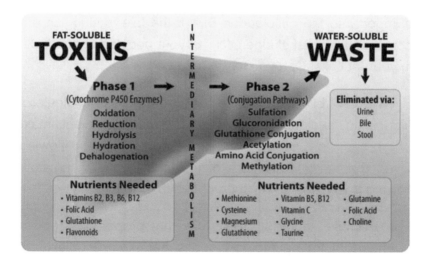

This harms your gallbladder as well. Your gallbladder is your liver's best friend. The liver secretes about a quart and half of bile daily, storing it in the gallbladder. When you eat fats, bile is released from your gallbladder into your intestine via the bile duct. Bile breaks down dietary fats into smaller particles that are more digestible and absorbable. A healthy gallbladder is essential for your body to absorb all the important fatty acids. It also helps you absorb fat-soluble vitamins such as vitamin A, vitamin E, vitamin K, and vitamin D. Fats are precursors to every hormone, so not digesting them has major consequences. If undigested fat globules pass from your gut into your bloodstream, your cells cannot incorporate them into cell membranes.

Your bile is also a magnet for toxins and everything the liver flushes out. These toxins then get stored in the bile and dumped into the gallbladder. But, if the bile is sluggish and congested, all that sludge sticks in your body and gets stored in your fat cells. Can you say, "Cellulite?"

Even worse, bile will become toxic from excess cholesterol, high toxin load, clogged bile ducts, and insufficient intake of the specific nutrients needed to keep it thin and flowing. Over time, the bile becomes toxic, thick, and sticky and stops flowing freely, and a multitude of health problems arise.

For example, many studies show that proper bile release is important for balancing blood sugar. Thicker bile leads to elevated blood sugar levels and bile acids are typically deficient in individuals with type-2 diabetes or insulin resistance.[3]

Thicker bile also leads to gallstone formation. One 2016 study published in the American Heart Association's journal *Arterioslcerosis, Thrombosis and Vascular Biology* showed that gallstones come with a 23% increased risk of coronary artery disease.[4] Moreover, gallbladder removal is the most frequently performed abdominal surgery in the United States today.

There's also a connection between toxic bile and a plethora of other chronic health conditions that negatively impact people's quality of life. Obesity is one. In an animal study, obese subjects secreted and released only half as much bile as did their leaner counterparts. Also, by the time people develop allergies, arthritis, and joint inflammation, they have a 75% bile deficiency. By the time they develop illnesses such as cancer or heart disease, their bile production is compromised by a whopping 90%.[5]

---

3   Gerald H. Tomkin and Daphne Owens, "Obesity diabetes and the role of bile acids in metabolism," *Journal of Translational Internal Medicine 4,* no. 2 (July 2016): 73–80, https://doi.org/10.1515/jtim-2016-0018.

4. Yan Zheng et al., "Gallstones and Risk of Coronary Heart Disease: Prospective Analysis of 270 000 Men and Women From 3 US Cohorts and Meta-Analysis," *Arteriosclerosis, Thrombosis, and Vascular Biology 36,* no. 9 (September 2016): 1997–2003, https://doi.org/10.1161/ATVBAHA.116.307507.

5   Ann Louise Gittleman, *Radical Metabolism: A Powerful New Plan to Blast Fat and Reignite Your Energy in Just 21 Days* (Boston, MA: Da Capo Lifelong Books, 2018).

My experience with my clients highlights the immense importance of having a healthy gallbladder and has led me to make some interesting observations about gallbladder dysfunction. First, I can't tell you how many women I've coached that don't have gallbladders or have had gallbladder stones. Second, I don't think that Western medicine or even fitness gurus spend enough time and effort on gallbladder health. When I think about the immense importance of the gallbladder, this makes no sense to me. As mentioned earlier, our liver is a powerful detoxification organ, but it takes an enormous beating from our toxic world. The same factors that have stressed our livers have dealt equally devastating blows to our gallbladder and bile flow. Third, the consequences of toxic bile go far beyond the inability to lose weight. The gallbladder breaks down all those fats you eat, which is critical for healthy cell membranes, and it helps cleanse your body of toxins. But, it also carries away hormone metabolites from your body. If your liver can't clean fats, it most likely cannot break down hormones or other metabolic waste products. Consequently, a sluggish thyroid could be a result of a clogged-up gallbladder. Finally, based on what I am seeing with my clients, it is time to think of unhealthy foods and lifestyle factors as being toxins that strain your liver, gallbladder, and bile. Refined sugar and grains, unhealthy fats, too little fiber, too much alcohol and caffeine, medications, and emotional stress are all quite hard on the liver and its companion organ, the gallbladder.

Toxin Overload

So, if our liver, gallbladder and bile are made for cleansing our bodies of toxins, why are they struggling to do so and, as a result, all this disease is occurring? The answer is simple. The toxic load is too great. According to the Environmental Protection Agency (EPA), we are being exposed to 86,000+ man-made chemicals every year. There is a daily assault on our bodies. We were not designed to filter out paint fumes, synthetic fragrances, plastics, and other man-made chemicals.

This is alarmingly evident in studies of umbilical cords. The umbilical cord supplies blood and nutrients to the unborn child. But it can often contain close to double the number of heavy metals, like mercury, than the mother contains in her own blood. In fact, umbilical cords of newborns typically contain over 100 toxins, cancer-causing chemicals, and heavy metals such as mercury, cadmium, and lead (11).[6]

Also, although it's not common knowledge, the world's leading health organizations have stated that 95% of all cancer is diet and environment-related (12).[7] It's no wonder our body continues to accumulate the toxicants it cannot convert into waste and stores them away in hopes of preventing harm to the internal organs. The body is extremely intelligent and

---

6   Stephen Cabral, *The Rain Barrel Effect: How a 6,000 Year Old Answer Holds the Secret to Finally Getting Well, Losing Weight & Feeling Alive Again!,* 1st ed. (CreateSpace Independent Publishing Platform, 2018), 24.

7   Cabral, *The Rain Barrel Effect.*

understands it can't store these toxins in your brain or heart because you'll die immediately. Instead, it stores them in your fat cells hoping that one day the liver will receive the right input of vitamins, minerals and nutrients while also having less of a toxic burden to deal with. But, trying so hard to eliminate these toxins is highly exhaustive for the liver and gallbladder. Think about it; they're bombarded by 86,000+ man-made chemicals a year! Over time, your body just becomes overwhelmed.

It is not easy to predict when your body will reach this point because every individual is different. Each person has their own limit or threshold and it is determined by a myriad of factors. Some of my mentors have referred to this as a "threat bucket." You can only pour so many "threats" into your bucket - environmental toxins, financial stress, relationship stress, poor sleep, poor diet/nutrition, etc, - until your bucket overflows and your body can no longer keep up with the toxic load. What determines your upper limit? Your age, genetics, gut microbiome, lifestyle, food intake, environmental exposures, etc. all play a role in what that level is for you.

Why Detox?

The liver and its companion organ, the gallbladder, exist to cleanse our bodies of chemical/biological toxins. But, this toxin overload means that they need some outside help to do their jobs. Remember, your liver is busy flushing out all the heavy metals, drugs, chemicals, pesticides, and preservatives you're being exposed to regularly. When your liver cannot keep up with the plastics, pesticides, heavy metals, and other chemicals in your blood, your body will look to force them out or store them in a "safe" place. Your body will actually push toxins through your skin. Think about that the next time you get eczema or some type of skin outbreak! When this doesn't work, your body prefers to store harmful chemicals in your fat cells with the hope of figuring out how to deal with those toxins later.

As a result, the weight gain issues we're facing in the present day have less to do with 'calories in and calories out' and 'exercising more.' Instead, our weight gain issues are driven by toxic foods, the hormonal and metabolic imbalances associated with exposure to chemical fragrances, soaps, deodorants, etc, and the toxin-heavy environment we live in.[8] This leads to an increase in inflammation and chemical storage in fat cells. This then leads to unnecessary water weight gain. Clients often confuse this toxic water weight with actual weight gain. That's why the 'calories in, calories out' approach doesn't just melt the weight off. As we know, some people eat far less than their friends but still can't manage to lose weight. I believe most of this is caused by this vicious cycle of toxicity.

So, why precisely is detoxing important when you're trying to lose weight? Well, let's start with some important facts: Fat cells make up what is referred to as adipose tissue. Our fat makes a great storage unit. Our blood shuttles toxins to our fat stores and then locks the door, sealing the toxins in that fat tissue.

---

8   Cabral, *The Rain Barrel Effect.*

Although this shields us from toxins and keeps us temporarily safe from immediate harm, there are consequences. We get fat. Literally, our adipose tissue begins to swell. You start to feel puffier, more swollen, and your body looks softer—like you're losing muscle tone.

Also, when these endotoxins build up in the body, a cascade of problems occurs: imbalanced gut bacteria, hormonal issues, a rise in inflammation and cortisol levels, and the accumulation of toxins directly deposited in your fat cells. This is why simply lowering your carbohydrate intake and exercising more will never get you to your goal of permanent weight loss.

Even more importantly, no one ever "just got an autoimmune disease." There's usually a series of events and toxic burdens (emotional and chemical) that trigger what modern doctors now call a certain disease such as lupus, multiple sclerosis, Alzheimer's, type 2 diabetes, etc. All of these "diseases" can be reversed as you soon as you rebalance the body and give it the correct input to heal.

Now, think of all the filters we have in our world, from our houses to our cars. Over time, all filters become dirty, congested, and clogged. Those filters must be changed every three to six months. It's the same thing with our bodies. Of course, we cannot just remove our organs and install new ones when they are getting dirty and clogged. Instead, we need to support our body's filtration system and open up our drainage/detox pathways. To this end, we must detoxify our livers and, in doing so, detoxify our gallbladders so that both organs can function optimally.

Liver Detox Basics

There are thousands of detoxes on the market, but the best way to detox is by *supporting* the liver, the main organ that cleanses your blood. I've studied under several naturopaths and functional medicine doctors over the last eight years and have had the chance to interview some top-level practitioners on my podcast. It's amazing how they all do things a little differently, but the principles are the same. When they start to heal clients' bodies, they focus on the liver and the drainage system of the body first before jumping into things like the gut microbiome and nervous system issues, etc. One of the most ancient forms of medicine, Ayurveda, understood this secret, and they detoxed the liver with certain herbs and amino acids. This practice is still used today.

The main idea of a liver detox is not to fill your body with lots of new supplements and vitamins or to add layers and layers of get-healthy products and technologies to your life – it is to give your body a few, carefully selected, natural products that will ignite your body's ability to heal itself. So, instead of supplementing with some new vitamin that you're deficient in, let's just remove the toxin that's creating the deficiency and allow the body to start making that needed nutrient like it's always known how to do. This is the crux of the liver detox.

You take what you know about how the liver works, then you give the body a few carefully selected tools that it will use to support the two main pathways of liver detoxification and then you enable the liver to detoxify itself.

It is also important to note that you also will need to help the body to help itself when you are working to detoxify your liver. A lot of built up toxins are going to be processed when you get your liver and gallbladder functioning better. You want to make sure that the waste created in the detoxification process is eliminated from your body in healthy ways. To this end, keeping the bowels moving (at first, you may need to add intestinal cleanses), sweating, resting and reducing stress can be helpful in your detoxification process.

TWO SUPPLEMENTS FOR LIVER DETOX THAT NO ONE TALKS ABOUT

Tudca

First of all, I'm a huge believer that when you do want or need to use supplements then you must use multiple supplements at once because it's the synergy of ingredients that makes the biggest difference. So, for me to tell you to take just one supplement and it'll change your life would normally be a ridiculous claim. However, the supplement Tudca is pretty magical, and there are many peer-reviewed studies to back that up. It's not widely known, but it is used heavily in the bodybuilding community because of its ability to support the liver and gallbladder and protect the liver and kidneys (bodybuilders are known for pumping their bodies with steroids and other supplements that are harsh on the liver and kidneys).

The other neat thing about Tudca is what the research says about insulin sensitivity and weight loss. Several studies are showing its efficacy with hyperglycemia associated with diabetes. In animal studies, Tudca has been shown to help lower blood sugar:

Animal studies indicate that TUDCA may help lower blood sugar. Type 1 diabetic animals received TUDCA for 24 days. After only 15 days, tests showed that their fasting blood sugar levels had lowered by 43%. In this study, researchers hypothesize the animals had more insulin because their pancreas cells started to produce insulin again.[9]

There are also multiple studies using Tudca to help regulate insulin resistance and up-regulate (to increase cellular activity) adiponectin. Adiponectin is a hormone that plays a huge role in insulin sensitivity as well as burning fat:

Treatment of obese and diabetic mice with these compounds resulted in normalization of hyperglycemia, restoration of systemic insulin sensitivity, resolution of fatty liver disease, and enhancement of insulin action in liver, muscle, and adipose tissues.[10]

---

9   Umut Özcan et al., "Chemical Chaperones Reduce ER Stress and Restore Glucose Homeostasis in a Mouse Model of Type 2 Diabetes," *Science 313*, no. 5790 (August 2006): 1137–1140, https://doi.org/10.1126/science.1128294.

10 Özcan et al., "Chemical Chaperones Reduce ER Stress."

Even more fascinating, the animal studies have shown that Tudca helps buffer cell stress and up-regulate the hypothalamus of offspring born to obese mothers. The hypothalamus is one of the major regulators of appetite and metabolism, so being able to up-regulate this part of the brain is huge.

In addition, the studies showed that Tudca supplementation had a myriad of other benefits. There were positive effects with hypertension, reducing blood pressure, and oxidative stress. There also were improved "metabolic and neurodevelopment deficits and reversed leptin resistance in the offspring." I've spoken several times about leptin resistance on my podcast. Leptin is a satiety-signaling hormone in our body that indicates fullness. Most people who are obese have disrupted leptin levels and eventually enter a stage of leptin resistance. Their brains stop getting the signal that it's satiated, and the cycle of overeating continues. Another win for Tudca!

Again, this is not a magical pill that makes you lose weight. But, it helps mobilize a sluggish gallbladder and protect and support the liver and kidneys. This will lead to downstream support for regulating hormones, cortisol levels, and blood sugar levels. Not only are the studies showing what it does for weight loss, but more importantly, for overall health. For all these reasons, I'm a huge fan of what Tudca can do. If you're interested in getting the Tudca I recommend for my clients, go to the resources section at the end of this chapter and the QR code will send you to a link of all my favorite resources listed in this book.

Lemon Essential Oil

I've been blessed to be surrounded by so many different holistic health practitioners over the last decade. I see how they get amazing results with getting their clients well, I study their different methodologies, and I continue to learn. One of the things I learned recently is that lemon essential oil can be great for detoxing and supporting the liver. Maybe you've heard people swear by the practice of squeezing some lemon in their morning cup of water with a pinch of salt to get their day going. It breaks down toxins or excess nutrients in the liver and eliminates those molecules via the kidneys and out of your body in your urine. There was even a great study done showing how citral, which is a component of the oil found in the peels of citrus fruits, was used to protect the liver against liver toxicity induced by high doses of acetaminophen.[11]

You can always squeeze a lemon into your water in the morning, but, as you can tell by now, I'm always looking for the edge and what can move the needle even more. I've seen amazing results with clients using a drop of doTerra's lemon essential oil in their glass of water in the morning. The essential oil is just way more concentrated and potent than fresh lemon juice, which is why I recommend it. It's also much easier to travel with than carrying a bag of lemons with you everywhere you go.

---

11   Nancy Sayuri Uchida et al., "Hepatoprotective Effect of Citral on Acetaminophen-Induced Liver Toxicity in Mice," *Evidence-Based Complementary and Alternative Medicine* (2017): 1796209, https://doi.org/10.1155/2017/1796209.

ACTION STEPS

1. **Do a Functional Medicine Detox:** I can't recommend enough a functional medicine detox to open those drainage pathways and support the liver. I've seen a lot of crap on the market, such as detox teas and juice cleanses, and, honestly, those don't work. I've even seen some 'influencers' selling expensive 3-day detoxes. It might work somewhat, but they're way overpriced, and it bothers me that they're using marketing to rip people off with the word "detox." If you're interested in learning more about functional medicine detoxes, as I believe they are one of the first things every person should do when they are on the road to health, please reach out to me and my team at *info@joelevancoaching.com*, and we'll be happy to get you setup.

2. **Take Detox Baby Steps:** If you're not going to try a full detox, just start with one thing that you can do. Maybe add a squeeze of lemon to your daily water, or buy one doTerra lemon essential oil and start adding that to your daily routine. Try taking Tudca. It's all about taking small steps and gaining small wins over time until those small wins compound into massive wins.

Avoid Toxins When Possible
Organic or Non-Organic Food?

I remember when the supermarket first started offering organic foods versus non-organic. The difference in prices bothered me, and I thought, "it's really not that big of a deal; I'll just go with the cheaper alternative…." Then, I read Senior MIT researcher Dr. Stephanie Seneff's book, *Toxic Legacy: How the Weedkiller Glyphosate Is Destroying Our Health & The Environment*. I also interviewed Dr. Seneff on my The Hacked Life podcast (Episode #107). Glyphosate is the name of the pesticide put into the infamous weed killer *Roundup* that has been sprayed on all our crops for years. We were told it was innocuous to humans and only killed the bugs trying to eat our crops. Well, research has found that not to be true.

Glyphosate is responsible for destroying so many pathways in our bodies: it destroys our ability to make glutathione (our master antioxidant), it destroys both the good bacteria in the gut microbiome and the tight junctions in the gut wall (which could then lead to autoimmune disorders), it destroys detox pathways such as the sulfur pathway, it hinders Vitamin D synthesis, it removes the body's ability to absorb glycine, an important amino acid responsible for the collagen matrix and bone health. There also is strong evidence to suggest that glyphosate causes neurological disorders, including autism.

Believe it or not, Glyphosate also can hinder your ability to lose weight. This happens in a couple of ways. First, it inhibits digestive enzymes in your body, such as lipase, which are responsible for breaking down fat cells. Second, there is strong evidence that it disrupts phosphoenolpyruvate carboxykinase (PEPCK), an enzyme that plays an essential role in gluconeogenesis by converting lactate, proteins, and fatty acids to glucose in the liver. PEPCK deficiency then affects the mitochondria which are the "power house" of all our cells except red blood cells. When this happens, PEPCK deficiency leads to, "a substantial decrease in activity and energy, a reduced number of muscle mitochondria, lower muscle mass, impaired ability of muscles to use fat as an energy source, and the accumulation of triglycerides in the blood, leading to their deposit into abdominal fat."[12] Furthermore, when PEPCK is disrupted in skeletal muscles, this leads to impaired utilization of lipids as a fuel source and reduction of the muscle's mitochondrial supply. This leaves the muscles impaired in their ability to perform sufficient exercise. Maybe we're not so lazy after all! Instead, we're being slowly poisoned by contaminated poor-quality food and overexposure to other persistent environmental toxicants.

Lastly, glyphosate has been shown to affect the liver. As you know, the liver is an extremely important filter for the body and the entire detoxification system. All the metrics used to assess impaired liver function have been found to be associated with glyphosate exposure in animal studies. Humans with liver disease have higher levels of glyphosate exposure in their urine than those with healthy livers. Even at doses below regulatory limits, Glyphosate caused fatty liver disease in rats. Fatty liver disease is an epidemic among humans today, even among young people.

---

12 Stephanie Seneff, *Toxic Legacy: How the Weedkiller Glyphosate Is Destroying Our Health and the Environment* (Vermont, USA: Chelsea Green Publishing, 2021), 113.

Consequently, I can't stress enough the importance of eating organic when you can. As I'm writing this book in the fall of 2022, inflation is through the roof, and food prices have skyrocketed. I get it, it's hard, and it's difficult to make ends meet, and we're all doing our best to provide for our families. If you can't eat organic all the time, I would definitely prioritize meats over fruits and vegetables. Also, you can prioritize where to put your money by following *The Clean 15* and *The Dirty Dozen*. *The Clean 15* is a list of foods you can eat that are less susceptible to pesticides and are, therefore, safer to purchase as non-organic. On the other hand, *The Dirty Dozen* is a list of foods that should always be purchased as organic because the non-organic versions are intensely sprayed with pesticides. Lastly, since moving to Idaho, we've made friends with many of our local organic farmers. It's been a wonderful experience, and I've learned that it is cheaper when I buy from them in bulk. I am very lucky to have access to this farm-fresh food. If at all possible, I encourage you to buy from farms, farmer's markets, etc.

To help you with deciding between organic and non-organic purchases, I have a PDF cheat sheet listed in my resources section when you scan the QR code below.

Most of these toxins are coming from tap, and especially bottled water, nearly invisible bits of polymer were also found in shellfish, beer, and salt, scientists and the University of Newcastle in Australia reported. The findings, drawn from 52 peer-reviewed studies, are the first to estimate the sheer weight of plastics consumed by individual humans: about 250 grams, or half-a-pound, over the course of a year.[13]

Another study calculated that the average American eats and drinks in about 45,000 plastic particles smaller than 130 microns annually while also breathing in roughly the same number of plastic particles.[14]

What's In Your Water?

"About 7.2 million Americans get sick every year from diseases spread through water."

-CDC

"Water hardness (inorganic minerals in solution) is the underlying cause of many, if not all, of the diseases resulting from poisons in the intestinal tract. These (hard minerals) pass

---

13 Kala Senathirajah and Thava Palanisami, "How Much Microplastics Are We Ingesting?: Estimation of the Mass of Microplastics Ingested," University News, The University of Newcastle, Australia, June 11, 2019, https://www.newcastle.edu.au/newsroom/featured/plastic-ingestion-by-people-could-be-equating-to-a-credit-card-a-week/how-much-microplastics-are-we-ingesting-estimation-of-the-mass-of-microplastics-ingested.

14 Kierna D. Cox, Garth A. Covernton, Hailey L. Davies, John F. Dower, Francis Juanes, and Sarah E. Dudas, "Human Consumption of Microplastics," *Environmental Science and Technology 53,* no. 12 (June 2019): 7068–7074, https://doi.org/10.1021/acs.est.9b01517.

from the intestinal walls and get into the lymphatic system, which delivers all of its products to the blood, which in turn, distributes to all parts of the body. This is the case of much human disease."

- Dr. Charles H. Mayo, Co-founder of the Mayo Clinic

You probably can't believe I'm actually going to talk about the type of water you drink in relationship to weight loss, but again, unlike many weight loss gurus, I don't look at this process in a 'calories in and calories out, eat less, and work out more' way. That's great for some, but I think we need to look at the body as a whole system. My goal always has been to get you healthy first, and then have weight loss happen as a natural by-product of this process. A big part of this 'get healthy and the weight loss will happen' process involves distilled water. It is the least toxic, purest form of water. It is water that has been boiled until it turns into vapor and is then converted back into liquid.

I learned about the power of distilled water from the practitioners in my circle who use it as a tool for helping their clients to heal from serious health issues such as autoimmune diseases like Lyme Disease and from mold toxicity. When these practitioners tested their clients, they noticed that radioactive chemicals and pesticides kept showing up in all of their clients. Interestingly enough, when the practitioners changed the water that their clients were drinking to distilled water, the clients started getting better rapidly. The levels of toxins in their clients dropped significantly and then their clients started pushing past their health plateaus.

If you're still not convinced, check out The Environmental Protection Agency's (EPA) website and see for yourself what we're up against. Remember, this agency is designed to oversee and protect Americans from harmful chemicals and toxins in our environment. Yet, they have flat-out told us on their website that 86,000+ manmade chemicals are bombarding you yearly. And that number is only increasing.

There are other sources of information pointing to the problems with environmental toxins including these two articles:

- "Ninety-eight percent of people in the U.S.A have measurable levels."[15]

- Evidence of microplastics found in human placenta.[16]

The article on microplastics stated:

Most of these toxins are coming from tap, and especially bottled water, nearly invisible bits of polymer were also found in shellfish, beer, and salt, scientists and the University of Newcastle in Australia reported. The findings, drawn from 52 peer-reviewed studies, are the first to estimate the sheer weight of plastics consumed by individual humans: about 250 grams, or half-a-pound, over the course of a year.

---

15 Brett Israel, "Widespread Plasticizer Clouds Doping Tests of Cyclists," *Scientific American,* February 9, 2021, https://www.scientificamerican.com/article/widespread-plasticizer-clouds-doping-tests-cyclists/.

16 Antonio Ragusa et al., "Plasticenta: First evidence of microplastics in human placenta," *Environmental International 146* (January 2021): 106274, https://doi.org/10.1016/j.envint.2020.106274.

Another study calculated that the average American eats and drinks in about 45,000 plastic particles smaller than 130 microns annually while also breathing in roughly the same number of plastic particles.[17]

Our water supply is also contaminated with radium – a radioactive chemical. This is not largely discussed or widely known. Health gurus do talk about contamination from heavy metals such as cadmium, mercury, and lead, and the general public is familiar with the dangers of lead poisoning in the home and with the issue of high mercury levels in certain seafood. But, what about radioactive chemicals? Unfortunately, many Americans are bombarded by radium, and they don't even know it. The Environmental Working Group (EWG) collected data from public water systems around the country and analyzed five years of tests from 2010 to 2015 and found radium in water supplies in all 50 states. The report showed 158 public water systems in 27 states "reported radium in amounts that exceeded the federal legal limit."[18] The result? Drinking water for more than 170 million Americans contains radioactive elements at levels that may increase the risk of cancer.

---

17 Julia Jacobo, "Humans consume the equivalent of a credit card worth of plastic every week: Report," abcNews, June 13, 2019, https://abcnews. go.com/US/humans-consume-equivalent-credit-card-worth-plastic-week/ story?id=63687144.

18 "170 Million in U.S. Drink Radioactive Tap Water," EWG.org, January 1, 2018, https://www.ewg.org/research/170-million-us-drink-radioactive-tap-water.

Why Water Distillation?

We've talked about how our "threat bucket" gets full over time, and eventually, that bucket starts to overflow. We're taking like 1,000 cuts a day from environmental toxins, radioactive elements, and pesticides on top of our daily stresses. So, if we can mitigate some of these cuts just by changing our water, wouldn't that be worth it? Give the body the right input, remove the toxicity creating the deficiencies in our systems, and our bodies will start to rebalance and heal.

There are many water purification systems on the market, and many of them are wonderful. But, at the end of the day, nothing removes impurities from our water as thoroughly as water distillation. Many of you will push back at me and say, "But Joel, what about the minerals you get from water!?" However, when it comes to water - and I've done a lot of research on this matter – humans have never relied heavily on getting minerals from our water. Instead, we get minerals from the food we eat.

Yes, minerals are hugely important. They are so important, in fact, that I add minerals (in the form of fulvic minerals) into my diet regularly. So, if you want more minerals, you can either supplement as I do (I will discuss this option more later in the book) or focus on eating a fully balanced, mineral-rich, nutritional diet. Most importantly, the ease of getting minerals from water does not balance out the danger of consuming those minerals alongside radium.

Also, check out my podcast (Episode #141) with the good folks at MyPureWater (my personal choice for home water distillation). We geek out on this topic and go into much more detail. Also, MyPureWater has patented dual vents on the cooling coil in their distillation system to vent off Volatile Organic Compounds (VOCs). If they condense down with the steam, the carbon filter in the system will get them. I've been using distilled water for over a year now with my family. We have only had positive results, and we haven't experienced any side effects or issues from switching to distilled water.

Why Not Reverse Osmosis (RO) Water?

RO water is great, but it's not better than distilled. Remember, 86,000+ man-made chemicals are bombarding us every year. How many impurities does RO remove? A recent Forbes article I found online said, "Even residential-grade reverse osmosis filters can remove up to 99% of lead, asbestos, and 82 other additional contaminants." So my question is, what about the other 85,918 contaminants? RO systems also lose effectiveness over time. Distillers are consistent, and they purify water by putting it through a 'phase change' instead of by passing it through a physical barrier. This means that whatever distillers remove the first time, they will remove the 1,000,000th time!

ACTION STEPS

1. **Learn More About Glyphosate:** The information I presented about glyphosate is just a small overview of the damage caused by this chemical. Please read Dr. Seneff's book *Toxic Legacy: How the Weedkiller Glyphosate Is Destroying Our Health & The Environment* and/or listen to Dr. Seneff on my The Hacked Life podcast (Episode #107) to learn more.

2. **Use The Clean 15 and The Dirty Dozen:** If it is not possible for you to buy all organic food, whether through lack of access to it or because of finances or both, you can still make a positive impact in lessening your toxin exposure by following these lists.

3. **Switch to Distilled Water:** I absolutely love the MyPureWater system. If you're interested in getting a MyPureWater system, go to their website, https://mypurewater.com, and use the code JOELEVAN for a discount. I'm glad that I found such a great American-made company that is filled with positive and hard-working folks.

Scan the QR code below to get a list of my go-to detox resources and a toxicity quiz to find out how toxic you really are.

Chapter 5

The Perfect Diet

You were not born a winner, and you were not born a loser. You are what you make yourself be.

-Lou Holtz

And now for diet – the easy part. Wait, what??? Diet is the hardest part of losing weight! Everyone knows that! Well, after you have developed the proper mindset, established clear values and visions for your goals, learned how to combat cravings, break bad habits and build good habits, worked on shedding the weight of negative emotions and traumas, and started to cleanse your body so that your organs function properly, diet becomes the fun part, the exciting part. You get to try new foods and feel invigorated by the foods you eat while you lose weight. Of course, 'easy' is a relative term. Nothing in life that is worth doing or having has ever come easy.

But, it is like you have been building a house from the ground up. You have cleared the lot, laid the foundation, built the framing, installed the wiring and plumbing, and put up the drywall. The infrastructure is in place, your house is solidly built and now you get to furnish it with the things you need to function on a daily basis. What's more, you get to select furnishings that appeal to you, that make you happy, and that help you to accomplish your daily needs and goals. These furnishings – these foods – will make your life and your body work well. Let your food be the fuel - the good, clean fuel - that ignites your energy and helps you to accomplish all your goals.

Diet Options

But, where to start? The options are overwhelming. One friend had success with this diet plan while another friend had success with that diet plan. You hear how miraculous someone feels on one diet or how another person's autoimmune problems disappeared on a completely different diet. The ads and commercials and messages are everywhere: Keto, Paleo, Carnivore, Mediterranean, Atkins, Weight Watchers, Nutrisystem, low-carb, low-fat, vegetarian, pescatarian, vegan …. and on and on.

Of the seemingly endless choices available these days, which is the perfect diet? It's impossible to say. Even though I like certain aspects of both Keto and Carnivore, there are pros and cons to each of these diets. I haven't reached the point where I can confidently say that doing either of those diets is the only thing I would ever do. As a matter of fact, I don't like saying, "I am Keto…" or "I am Carnivore…" I think it limits you at that very moment from the possibility of learning anything new. Once you take on the identity of something, it makes it difficult to take in new information, even if it might save your health.

Now I know many of you will say, "But Joel, what about Atkins, low-carb, Weight Watchers, vegan, etc. ….? Interestingly enough, studies have shown that people who actually maintain weight loss long-term aren't succeeding because they all happen to have found the same perfect, specific diet. Instead, they are succeeding because they found the diet that works for them, and they are able to stick to that diet long-term. This diet will be different for different individuals. To this end, I think most people should experiment and see what works for them in the long run. Test, experiment, retest, and see what works best for you based on your bio-individuality.

Principles of the Weight Loss Diet

There are, however, some fundamentals that can guide you in your quest to find the diet that enables you to meet your weight loss goals, makes you feel well-fueled and energized, and works for you long-term.

1. Keep in mind the information I provided in the last chapter about the benefits of eating organic foods whenever possible and drinking distilled water, and then integrate that knowledge into how you eat and hydrate.

2. Try to fast for a minimum of 12 hours every day. This is not as daunting as it seems because the fasting time overlaps with your sleeping time. As with your diet, you will need to experiment with what works best for you based on your bio-individuality. Ideally, you will fast for at least 12 hours. But, maybe for you, it needs to be 8 or 10 hours. Or, maybe, 14, 15 or 16 hours will work best for you.

3. Understand the diets of people who live in places around the world where there is less suffering from weight-related issues.

For number 3, there are some key, overarching themes that emerge from an analysis of the foods and eating habits of people who live in places where obesity and its attendant health issues are less of a problem than here in America. This information has been gathered, analyzed, and written about by both Dr. Catherine Shanahan and Dr. Daphne Miller. Taken together, it is my belief that their research establishes the best practices for a weight loss diet.

Dr. Catherine Shanahan, who was the sports nutritionist for the Los Angeles Lakers when they won many titles, is the author of *Deep Nutrition*: *Why Your Genes Need Traditional Food*. In this book, Dr. Shanahan outlines what her research shows to be 'The Four Pillars' of the human diet.

The Four Pillars are:

- Meat on the bone
- Fermented and sprouted foods
- Organs and other "nasty bits"
- Fresh, unadulterated plant and animal products

Dr. Shanahan came up with these 'The Four Pillars' after doing extensive research on diets from all around the world. She analyzed those diets, figured out which diets have proven to help people live longer, healthier lives and then condensed those diets into these four, fundamental commonalities.

Similar to Dr. Shanahan's work, Dr. Daphne Miller also looked at the healthiest diets from around the world and analyzed why they work and how to make them work for us. She compiled all of her research into her book, *The Jungle Effect: A Doctor Discovers the Healthiest Diets from Around the World and How to Bring Them Home.* Dr. Miller was inspired to conduct her research because she wanted to understand why her patients of certain ethnicities, who had thrived on diets when they were in their homelands, were much less healthy when they were eating the Americanized versions of their native diets. Dr. Miller traveled to many of the regions where her patients had come from in order to learn why and how the indigenous foods and diet had prevented all the chronic and common diseases her patients were suffering from now. Like Dr. Shanahan, Dr. Miller condensed her findings into some guiding principles. Her book outlines what she found to be the nine core principles of an indigenous diet. The result is:

The Anatomy of an Indigenous Diet: The 9 Key Components

1. Foods that are local, fresh, and in season

2. Food cultivation techniques and recipes passed down through the ages

3. Food traditions:
   a. Communal eating
   b. Eating for satiety rather than fullness
   c. Observation of fasts and other food rituals

4. Sugar from whole foods such as honey, fruits, vegetables, and whole grains

5. Salt from natural, unprocessed sources such as fish, sea greens, and vegetables

6. Naturally raised meat and dairy as a precious commodity:
   a. Meat and dairy in small quantities to complement vegetables, whole grains, and legumes
   b. Organ meats and whey used in cooking
   c. Liberal use of proteins from non-meat sources such as nuts, legumes, and whole grains

7. Non-meat fats from whole nuts, seeds, grains, and fatty fruits; minimally processed oils such as olive, palm fruit, or coconut oil

8. Fermented and pickled foods

9. Healing spices

You can see there's some nice cross-over between both Dr. Shanahan's 'The Four Pillars' and Dr. Miller's 'The 9 Key Components.' Both are advocating for less processed food and more fresh food while utilizing ancient techniques such as sprouting and fermentation. I think both 'The Four Pillars' and 'The 9 Key Concepts" are generally good recommendations and their principles should be utilized by anyone looking for a balanced, healthy long-term diet plan.

Note: I know people reading this book who might be vegans or vegetarians will feel like most of 'The Four Pillars' and parts of 'The 9 Key Components' cannot offer them any guidance in choosing their perfect weight loss diet. I'm not here to disagree with you or prove that your idea about the perfect diet is wrong. I personally think 'The Four Pillars' and 'The 9 Key Components' are some really good principles and make sense overall for the majority of people. Moreover, I work with many vegans and vegetarians, and we still get great results following similar principles, but we use tailored supplementation to make up for the benefits of eating meat. At the end of the day, though, you need to do what's right for your ethics and your biology.

The Foundation of All Diets

The Four Pillars' and 'The 9 Key Components" certainly offer a wealth of guidance for what and how to eat as well as how to prepare food. Through my studies and certifications, I've narrowed the overarching principles down even further and created specific categories, percentages, and amounts as a guide for putting together a daily diet. Of course, individual needs and circumstances may necessitate different requirements, but, in general, your daily food intake should be broken down as follows:

Fruits & Vegetables

More specifically, 60% - 80% of all your food intake should be plant-based and should be predominately vegetables. No food nourishes the body in more ways than plants and fruits. Plants and fruits contain phytonutrients, enzymes, antioxidants (vary with color), fiber, vitamins, minerals, and the amino acids and proteins that are the building blocks of life. They are nutrient-dense, living foods that are unprocessed and non-cancer-causing and are mainly composed of water. They also are easy to digest.

Note: Some people have difficulty digesting certain plants. These people generally suffer from a condition called gut dysbiosis. This is an imbalance of the gut microbiome, and it causes a host of GI issues such as leaky gut. People with this disorder are unable to break down some plant compounds and this exacerbates their leaky gut even more. If you have problems tolerating and digesting certain plants, I would run an organic acids test and connect with a health practitioner like myself or a holistic doctor who can interpret these labs to give you a better understanding of what's going on with your gut and other detox pathways.

The Weight Loss Diet Plan

75% Vegetables
25% Protein
2 TBSP of Fat

Notice I didn't mention fruits here even though I listed several reasons why fruit is extremely hydrating and good for you. In the beginning of your weight loss journey, I would not recommend eating high amounts of fruit since fruit is a sugar. Instead, I recommend limiting your fruit intake for the first three weeks of your diet and then slowly reintroducing it and seeing how your body reacts. I will share with you what I do for maintenance purposes, but, in general, this is the macro blueprint for success when it comes to losing weight.

Getting Started

1. I highly recommend everyone go through some type of functional liver detox to start. This is going to help open those drainage pathways, purify your body and blood, and prep your body for what's to come (I personally take my clients through a 3-week detox).

2. After completing a detox, I allow my clients one FlexMeal or "cheat meal" a week (Yes, I just said "cheat meals." I have not discussed them in this chapter, but you and I both know they are a reality. Total deprivation will only backfire. Instead, be very smart and very judicious in your "cheat meals." Also, spreading them out and choosing them wisely will not only help your health and your weight loss goals, but doing so will enable you to savor them more).

3. Add fruit to one meal (Ex. breakfast smoothie).

4. Then add a starch at lunch (½ cup).

5. Stop adding fruit/starch when weight loss plateaus.

6. If you're still not at your desired weight loss, consider completing another detox.

I Practice What I Preach

To turn all these concepts, percentages and measurements into something more concrete and serviceable, I will share what I do for my daily diet. This is the same diet that also works for most of my clients.

Before getting started, though, here are a few quick tips and practices that help me and my clients stay on track with our daily diets.

- No snacking
- Drink plenty of water (1/2 your body weight in ounces)

- Walk after meals (especially dinner)
- Plan meals in advance
- Fast 12-16 hours each day
- Spread out your cheat meals 48-72 hours apart to limit inflammation

Breakfast

I recommend that most of my clients begin their day with a smoothie. They are my breakfast of choice as well. I like smoothies because they are easier to digest than other, more typical, breakfast foods. This is important because, for most people, their digestion is wrecked, and they can't break down food all the way. These digestion problems are compounded by high loads of stress, lack of sleep, being constantly on the go, and having no time for making breakfast. Additionally, 30% of all your energy goes to digestion! So, if we can find ways to get more energy back into our day, wouldn't that be helpful?

Plus, when we wake up in the morning, we are extremely dehydrated after our bodies have been lying down stagnant for multiple hours, and, for many of us, one of the first things we do is to reach for a cup of coffee (I do too, so no judgment). Unfortunately, though, coffee is dehydrating. Instead, we need to rehydrate the body. Smoothies help rehydrate the body. They also contain the vitamins and minerals needed to energize and flush the body.

My Personal Smoothie

- 20-30 oz of distilled water
- 1/2-1 cup of frozen organic blueberries
- Knob of ginger (I add this mostly in winter to bring heat to the body and aid in digestion.)
- Nutritional Multivitamin/Multimineral Powder
- Fulvic minerals (There is more information about fulvic minerals at the end of this book.)
- Ceylon Cinnamon (I add it for taste and because it is a powerful polyphenol that helps with insulin sensitivity. My personal favorite is Anthony's.)
- Olive oil (1 TBSP) or MCT oil (1 TBSP)
- 1 cup of greens (fresh organic spinach or Power Greens)
- Sometimes I'll also add one drop of doTerra's MetaPWR blend (It contains cinnamon for blood sugar regulation, lemon/grapefruit oil to support detox, and peppermint/ginger to stimulate thermogenesis.)

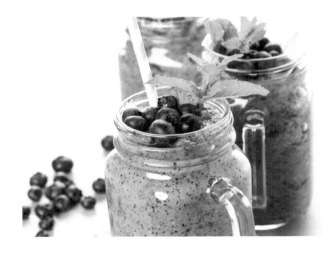

Lunch

For most of my lunches, I simply make myself a salad with cucumbers, baby carrots, and pumpkin seeds (for crunch and extra zinc, selenium, and magnesium). I then add salt and olive oil. Then, depending on my mood and needs, I may add some type of protein like eggs, an organic sausage, sardines, chicken breast, etc. You also can add plant-based protein sources if you're vegan, like hemp seeds or tofu. Most of the time, that's it. That is my lunch. It is also the lunch I recommend for my clients.

If people find it too boring, I recommend adding balsamic vinegar or extra herbs like basil, cilantro, or oregano to the salad. You also could add sauerkraut for a healthy probiotic. But, if you still find it too boring even with those additions, you could try a healthy salad dressing. The only brand I can recommend is Primal Kitchen. They make wonderful salad dressings that use avocado oil as the base and are quite tasty and healthy.

Finally, you also could add 1/2-1 avocado for a good clean fat and to help improve satiety and fullness. I do find that extra protein keeps me and my clients satiated longer in between meals, and we don't feel the need to snack between lunch and dinner. But, if I'm protein-fasting or limiting my intake of animal products for some reason, then using the avocado helps keep me satiated between lunch and dinner.

Weight Loss Lunch Guidelines

- 2 cups of vegetables (raw or cooked)
- 0-1 cup of root vegetables (sweet potato, yucca, squash, etc.)
- 1/2-1 cup (3.5 - 6 oz.) of protein (vegan/paleo etc.)
- 1-2 TBSP of healthy fat (olive oil or smashed avocado)
- Spices (oregano, cayenne, parsley, rosemary, etc.)

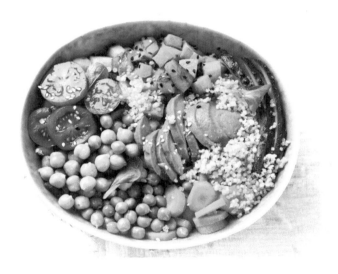

I Need More Variety!

I feel like I have an abundance of variety in my diet, but, if you notice, my breakfast and lunch are more or less the same every day. There are some minor variations here and there, but I stick with my smoothie for breakfast and my salad for lunch. This is very intentional.

You'd think having more choices would give you better options for healthier food choices. But, the fact is that too many options lead to indecision and this, in turn, leads to bad choices. One of the hallmarks of success among entrepreneurs and busy professionals is being decisive and taking action. Over the last nine years, I've been a husband and dad, managed a side business, and worked over 60 hours weekly in my regular job. I've also worked with many clients who are busy professionals who are similarly short on time. Adding more variety and choices into their busy schedules only confuses them and creates the "paradox of choice."

By maintaining a regular, consistent breakfast and lunch for the last nine years, I avoid all that noise. I avoid brain fatigue by taking away the "I wonder what I'll have for breakfast and lunch today...?" dilemma. I already know. It's scheduled. It's automatic. It's the same thing we see with some of the most successful people in the financial world. Most millionaires aren't great because they invested in some IPO stock or made millions off crypto. Instead, they have automated their investing.

Dinner

By having similar meals for breakfast and lunch, you only need to focus on figuring out a healthy dinner. My wife and I have made healthy dinners for our family of four for over nine years. We are able to do it easily and consistently because we keep it simple. We know, in general, that our dinner will follow some of the principles I've already outlined in this chapter. It will most likely have a starch, a vegetable, and a protein.

We stick to a consistent array of healthy starches to eliminate decision fatigue: white rice, baked sweet potatoes/Japanese sweet potatoes, and baby white/red potatoes. All these starches are easy to make in an oven or InstaPot. We just "set it and forget it," and then start making our vegetables and protein. For veggies, we stick to mostly broccoli, Brussel sprouts, green beans, and asparagus. I don't have much of a background in cooking, but even I can quickly throw these in a pan with olive oil, salt, turmeric, and garlic powder and make them taste flavorful. As for proteins, we always purchase organic, grass-fed meat, and it's either grilled, thrown in a crock pot, or done in the pan.

I promise you, the more you start cooking regularly, the easier it becomes. Our meals typically last us for two nights (I do not recommend cooking for more than three nights at a time due to bacteria growing on food). That means you only need to cook about three times a week, and, if you're doing the plan right, the only meal you have to plan for is dinner, which makes this *diet* sustainable and long-lasting. Remember, there are plenty of studies showing that the diet you can adhere to consistently is the most effective diet.

Weight Loss Dinner Guidelines

- 2+ cups of vegetables (raw or cooked)
- No root vegetables for the first 3 weeks (you can add one more cup of vegetables or use sprouts or 1/2 avocado)
- 1/2-1 cup (3.5 - 6 oz.) of protein (vegan/paleo, etc.)
- 1-2 TBSP of healthy fat (olive oil or smashed avocado)
- Spices (oregano, cayenne, parsley, rosemary, etc.)

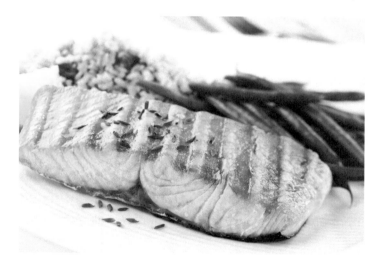

To get my free Weight Loss Diet Cheat Sheet and Meal Plan as well as my Healthy Shopping List, scan the QR code below.

If You're Still Hungry In Between Meals

If you are just too hungry between meals to avoid snacking, there are several issues that could be driving your hunger:

1. **Dehydration**. You could be dehydrated and need more water. Try drinking more water 30 minutes before your next meal or one hour after eating a meal.

2. **Mineral Deficiency**. You might also be mineral deficient and need more salt and electrolytes. Try adding an electrolyte powder, such as LMNT, to your water. LMNT was created by health pioneer Robb Wolff and is sugar free, Keto and Paleo friendly, etc. For another mineral supplement option, I am a huge fan of adding fulvic minerals to my water. One of my favorite brands is BEAM Minerals.

3. **Insufficient Protein Intake**. If adding more water and minerals to your diet doesn't improve satiety, try adding more protein to your meals to improve fullness.

4. **Underlying Issues**. If none of these help, you could be eating inflammatory foods that are causing reactions in your body. You could run a Food Sensitivity Test. You also may need to consult a functional medicine practitioner in order to perform a functional medicine detox so that you can help reset your body.

ACTION STEPS

1. **Have a Plan:** Plan your shopping and plan your meals. Download my *Shopping List* and my *Weight Loss Diet Cheat Sheet and Meal Plan.*

2. **Do Your Research:** With so many options for diets, you need to educate yourself about the possibilities. At the very least, read Dr. Shannahan's and Dr. Miller's books.

3. **Fast:** Aim to fast for a minimum of 12 hours out of every day. If you can do more, great. If you cannot, then fast for at least 8 hours.

4. **Variety is Not Always the Spice of Life:** Start every day by having a smoothie for breakfast. Then have a mostly plant-based lunch (add protein if needed). Your dinner will be your most varied meal of the day although it should still follow the same ratio of starch, vegetable and protein every night.

5. **Keep a Food Journal:** In order to get an idea of how often you're eating, what you are eating and what foods might be causing an inflammatory response in your body (bloating, digestion issues, fatigue, brain fog, skin issues, etc.), keep an honest and thorough accounting of all that you eat.

Chapter 6

Exercise/Movement

Exercise is like brushing your teeth. It is good for you and should be done every day. Just don't expect to lose weight.

-Dr. James Fung

Finally! It's time to talk about the need for exercise in your weight loss program. Well, if that's what you are thinking, then hold onto your hat…. this chapter is going to shock you because I am here to tell you that neither cardio nor long workouts are the key to weight loss. Yes, you read that right! In fact, the purpose of this chapter is to tell you two important things that will help you achieve your weight loss goals:

1. Cardio is a Waste of Time for Weight Loss

2. You Can Effectively Workout in Just 10 Minutes a Day

This is great news for all you folks who have consistently exercised and still haven't lost a single pound. The fact that exercise produces less weight loss than expected has been well-documented in medical research. Long-term studies that lasted twenty-five weeks or more found that exercise led to a weight loss that was only 30% of what study participants expected. For example, in a recent 10-month-long controlled study, some participants increased their exercise to five times per week, burning 600 calories per session. In doing so, they expected to lose about 35 pounds. They did not, and they only lost an average of one pound more than the study participants who were not following the same increased exercise protocol.

So Why Even Exercise?

Well, keeping in mind the metaphor we previously used to equate your weight loss journey with building a house from the ground up, exercise is the equivalent of decorating that house. You've created the foundation, the structure, and the infrastructure and you have put in place the furnishings that you need to function on a daily basis. Now, you get to put in the pieces that are good for your mind, body, and soul. This décor can change with time and seasons, it can be elaborate or minimalist or anywhere in between, and it can vary greatly from that of your neighbors and friends. But, in general, it is what makes you feel happy and comfortable in your 'house.' It adds positive energy to your life.

Exercise, for me and most of my clients, does so much more than help you to lose weight. Although you associate exercise with being good for your muscles, exercise is actually very good for your brain as well. Exercise is known to have numerous neuroprotective and cognitive benefits, especially in memory and learning-related processes. Although the precise mechanisms of this link are not fully understood, it is known that exercise increases brain-derived neurotrophic factor (BDNF). In a nutshell, neurotrophins are proteins that keep your nervous system healthy. As a member of the neurotrophin family, BDNF regulates many of the processes within neurogenesis - the formation of new neurons in the brain. In terms of the hippocampus, the area of the brain responsible for learning and memory, BDNF is responsible for hippocampal neurogenesis. It is through this link between exercise and increased BDNF that it is possible for exercise to improve cognition. Exercise-mediated hippocampal neurogenesis, which generates new neurons and incorporates them into hippocampal circuits, improves your ability to learn and remember.[19]

Interestingly enough, there's some evidence to suggest that exercise also improves satiety signals in the brain. In other words, regular exercise improves your appetite regulation at a neural level. This is extremely important for weight loss because a dysregulation in the body's ability to feel "full" will lead to over-eating. Long-term weight loss studies show that most people who don't do well with weight loss suffer from an imbalance of leptin and gherkin, the hormones

19 Adrián De la Rosa et al., "Long-term exercise training improves memory in middle-aged men and modulates peripheral levels of BDNF and Cathepsin B," *Scientific Reports 9,* no. 3337 (March 2019), https://doi.org/10.1038/s41598-019-40040-8.

that regulate appetite.[20] The studies also show that when people supplemented with peptides such as semaglutide, an appetite regulator, they could maintain long-term weight loss successfully.

My personal experience backs up these studies. I've experimented with a lot of fasting throughout the years and found that low-to-moderate intensity exercise has helped me to stave off feeling hungry during my fasting times. It makes me feel fuller longer, and I don't even think about wanting food. Exercise also helps me stay consistent with healthy eating. When I exercise, I prioritize eating healthy to fuel my body. It acts as an anchor and reminder to fuel my body with good stuff, not junk. I've never finished a workout and thought, "Oh, perfect, now I can eat a chocolate cake." Since appetite regulation and control are huge for long-term weight loss success, and you can use something free like exercise to improve them, you should invest!

Lastly, exercise improves your health by increasing insulin sensitivity and lowering inflammation and oxidative stress. It is well established "that acute exercise is associated with substantial improvement in insulin sensitivity. A single bout of moderate-intensity exercise can increase the glucose uptake

---

20 Public Library of Science, "Exercising restores sensitivity of neuron that make one feel full," ScienceDaily,, August 25, 2010, https://www.sciencedaily. com/releases/2010/08/100824171614.htm#:~:text=Besides%20burning%20 calories%2C%20exercise%20restores,intake%20and%20consequently%20 weight%20loss.

by at least 40%."[21] So, even if the exercise you are doing is not making you lose weight, it is improving your overall health and lowering inflammation biomarkers.

Mitochondria

The benefits of exercise go even deeper than neurons and hormones. Exercise benefits your body at the intra-cellular level. It actually helps your body to make energy. Now, you might be thinking, "It takes a lot of energy to exercise. Exercise wears me out. How is that *making* energy?" In order to reconcile this seeming contradiction, you have to understand the mitochondria.

For simplification purposes, mitochondria are known as the "powerhouses of our cells." They are tiny organelles that exist in the hundreds to thousands within every cell of our bodies except our red blood cells. Within these little "power plants," the glucose and fatty acids that come from our food are converted into the form of energy that our body needs to work. This energy is called ATP (adenosine triphosphate), and it is the fuel that powers our organs.

Like man-made power plants, these cellular energy producers can wear out over time. However, unlike a human-built power

---

21 Vighnesh Vetrival Venkatasamy, Sandeep Pericherla, Sachin Manthuruthil, Shikha Mishra, and Ram Hanno, "Effect of Physical activity on Insulin Resistance, Inflammation and Oxidative Stress in Diabetes Mellitus," *Journal of Clinical & Diagnostic Research 7,* no. 8 (July 2014): 1764–1766, https://doi.org/10.7860/JCDR/2013/6518.3306.

plant, it is relatively easy to create new mitochondria. Exercise helps to stimulate the creation of new mitochondria. It also helps your existing mitochondria to work more efficiently. This is pretty amazing stuff – you use some energy to exercise and your body rewards you with the creation of more energy and better energy!

This exercise and mitochondria duet occurs in our fat cells as well. In our bodies, we have two types of fat: white fat and brown fat. White fat, also known as visceral fat, is the kind of fat everyone wants to get rid of (and is deadly for your health). It is made up of fatty acids, and it is where our bodies store extra calories (energy it isn't using). Brown fat is a more specific and less abundant form of fat in our bodies. It produces heat to help maintain our body temperature in cold conditions. Brown fat is much more mitochondrial-dense than white fat because it needs a lot of "power plants" to burn calories in order to produce body heat. Interestingly, research is showing that exercise may stimulate hormones that activate brown fat and that brown fat appears to be able to use white fat as fuel. This is definitely a win-win!

Understanding the importance of our mitochondria also highlights that it is essential to keep our "power plants" as healthy as possible. This is particularly evident when you understand that your mitochondria are critical when it comes to insulin secretion. Your body makes insulin in its beta cells. These beta cells not only produce insulin, they also must produce and release the right amount of insulin at the right time. Releasing too much can result in life-threatening hypoglycemia, and releasing too little results in high blood glucose. So, the hundreds to thousands of mitochondria inside each of your beta cells must be functioning at optimal levels in order for these all-important cells to do their job well.

When this delicate balance is upset, the results are profoundly bad for your health and well-being. Researchers know that having dysfunctional mitochondria leads to insulin resistance, and they also know that insulin resistance can lead to mitochondrial dysfunction. There is deliberation over *which came first,* but, either way, being insulin insensitive means that the cells in your muscles, fat, and liver don't respond well to insulin. They can't easily take up glucose from your blood. This problem is at the heart of many metabolic disorders. In addition, dysfunctional mitochondria lead to autoimmune conditions, chronic fatigue, etc.

As you can see, having strong, healthy mitochondria is a big deal when managing metabolic disease and chronic disease in general, and exercise is key to keeping the mitochondria healthy. In addition, regular, daily exercise can significantly reduce the amount of insulin necessary to control your blood glucose. This lessens the work load of your beta cells which, in turn, keeps their mitochondria from wearing out. These mitochondria are then in better condition to convert glucose into energy.

Consequently, optimal mitochondrial functioning is like the saying, "You need money to make money." Exercise helps your mitochondria to be healthy so that your organs can function properly. Then, when your organs are functioning well, your mitochondria are healthier and they help you to exercise. Therefore, making that exercise investment in healthy mitochondria pays dividends in your overall health and well-being.

But What Kind of Exercise Should You Do?

I meet so many clients who tell me how often they are in the gym and all the cardio they are doing, and the first thing I'm thinking is, "No wonder you're not losing weight. Why are you doing cardio?" Cardio is great for selling *Muscle & Fitness* magazines, but it doesn't trigger weight loss. In fact, cardio stimulates cortisol, your natural stress hormone.

When I interviewed Dr. John Jaquish, founder of the X3 Bar, co-founder of the OsteoStrong company, and best-selling co-author of *Weightlifting Is A Waste of Time,* he said that cortisol undermines your fitness in two ways. First, cortisol has the potential to inhibit lipolysis which, in basic terms, is the breaking down of fat. Cortisol, therefore, protects body fat. Second, cortisol can promote proteolysis, which, simply put, is the breakdown of proteins. Through this process, cortisol leads to the breakdown of lean muscle tissue. Furthermore, Dr. Jaquish explains in his book that "doing hours of cardio tells the body that it needs to go long distances with a limited amount of fuel. It responded by protecting that fuel, holding onto fat as long as possible."[22]

Right now, you might be full of questions: "So now what?" "Should I stop doing cardio altogether?" "What if I like doing cardio?" Or, "Yay! I hate doing cardio. Can I stop it and never, ever do it again?" Well, there are benefits to doing limited cardio-oriented workouts. In fact, I still include some cardio in my exercise regimen because cardio has still been found to be beneficial for you overall longevity and cardiovascular system. Studies show that moderate intensity cardio helps your cells clear out old, malfunctioning mitochondria through a process called mitophagy.[23] And, remember, healthy mitochondria is a hallmark of aging. Just don't expect that your cardio exercise will have a direct connection to weight loss.

Instead, for weight loss, focus on the exercises that have a positive effect on growth hormone and testosterone because these major hormones are responsible for weight loss and muscle gain. The question, then, is, "What triggers the release of growth hormone and testosterone?" The answer is: resistance training, i.e., body weight exercises, weight training, and/or resistance band training. In other words, you need to exercise and strengthen your muscles in order to lose weight.

---

22 Dr. John Jaquish and Henry Alkire, *Weight Lifting Is a Waste of Time: So Is Cardio, and There's a Better Way to Have the Body You Want* (Carson City, Nevada: Lioncrest Publishing, 2020), 49.

23 Jonathan M Memme, Avigail T. Erlich, Geetika Phukan, and David A. Hood, "Exercise and mitochondrial health," *Journal of Physiology 599,* no. 3 (November 2019): 803–817, https://doi.org/10.1113/JP278853.

Muscle, like brown fat, is an innate energy burner. In fact, for every pound of muscle tissue, you will burn 50 calories daily, whereas, for every pound of white fat, you will burn only 2 calories daily. Also, like in brown fat, mitochondria are densely packed in your muscle tissues. Each muscle cell contains thousands of mitochondria. Muscle mitochondria are mainly responsible for generating the ATP, or energy, needed to control how nutrients get in and out of the muscle cells and to contract and elongate muscle fibers when you exercise.

When you challenge your muscle to contract regularly through movement and exercise, muscle fibers respond to the force by creating more mitochondria to burn more fuel and process more oxygen the next time they are required to perform work. So, if you want to make more mitochondria in your muscle tissue, all you need to do is exercise. Then, when you do exercise, mitochondria can increase ATP production by as much as 100 times. This is why regular muscle strengthening and building exercises improve your endurance, strength, and overall ability to perform work.

How Muscle Really Grows

As a young kid, I was taught that you need to tear the muscle by lifting heavy weights in order for it to regrow, get stronger, and get bigger. But, when I interviewed Dr. Sam Buckner from the University of Florida Muscle Laboratory, a doctor specializing in muscle growth, he told me that wasn't entirely true. He explained that you don't need to tear the muscle for it to grow; you simply need to exhaust the muscle to failure (full fatigue) so that a cell-signaling response leads to metabolic adaptations in the musculature that will cause it to grow later. In other words, resistance training as well as high-intensity exercise creates the protein cascade that initiates the protein synthesis which causes muscle growth.

But, is high-intensity the same thing as heavy-weight training? Dr. Buckner conducted studies looking at low-load training vs. heavy-load training (i.e., light weights vs. heavy weights) and found that they both produce muscle growth. The heavy load training, however, was associated with more muscle damage. This led Dr. Buckner to believe that muscle damage was not needed to facilitate actual muscle growth.

Dr. Buckner even conducted a study using "no-load training," meaning the participants were not using any weights to build muscle. He wanted to see if, for example, simply flexing the bicep while using internal tension was enough to build muscle versus the typical four sets of 12 repetitions schema we've all been taught. What he found was that muscle growth was similar in both conditions. That study proved that you don't need external load (i.e., weights) to grow a muscle. You need stress and tension to activate those muscle fibers.

So, what is the best way to exercise that will stress (not tear) your muscles so that they will strengthen and grow? Based on the research and data, it appears that variable resistance training (resistance band training) is king. Variable resistance offers more of an anabolic output than regular weight training. Furthermore, research supports an increased hormonal response through variable resistance training compared to weightlifting. For example, in one study, all participants were measured both pre- and post-experiment for testosterone and growth hormone. During the study, all of the participants performed the same exercise protocol. But, some used resistance bands, and others used weights. Results showed that the variable resistance group using bands experienced a greater increase in both testosterone and growth hormone than those performing traditional weightlifting.[24]

That said, if you love doing weights, by all means, continue to do weights. However, you have to use a weight where you are unable to continue repetitions after thirty to sixty seconds.

Also, during our interview, I asked Dr. Buckner if he feels that completing one set of exercises to failure is enough to stimulate muscle growth, which is what Dr. Jaquish advocates. Dr. Buckner stated that it definitely is possible. However, his recommendation is to perform two sets to failure to ensure that all the muscle fibers are fully exhausted and that a cell-signaling response is created. Whether you opt for completing one set or two sets to failure, it is important to appreciate where you are in your physical fitness journey. You may achieve full fatigue through exercise that is somewhat intense. However, exercise that is highly-intense will reap the

---

24   aquish and Alkire, 57.

most benefits. Therefore, it could become a goal for you if you are not already there.

So, whether you opt for resistance bands or weights, you should adopt the following protocol:

The Minimum Effective Dose For Exercise

1. Perform one to two sets to failure for each exercise. 60-120 seconds of total time under tension per exercise.

2. Use a 5/5 Rep Cadence (5 seconds up, 5 seconds down). You can do 2/2 or even 3/3; however, slow and controlled elicits more stability firing, which will elicit a greater growth hormone response.

3. Focus on 2-10 different exercises per workout.

Is 10 minutes a Day of Exercise Really enough?

Now that we know that high-intensity and variable resistance training, or, if you prefer, high-intensity weight training, are actually the best ways to stimulate the hormones that help with weight loss, we have to examine how much time we need to put into that training. With most of my clients, going to the gym is difficult, and they don't have time in their day. So, the more you can do in the least amount of time is always a win.

But, this is the beauty of high-intensity training – it is the form of exercise that is best for strengthening and building your muscles and helping you to lose weight, and it also is the form of exercise that only takes minutes out of your day. In fact, look at the protocol above. We are measuring your exercises in seconds, not minutes or hours. There is no more need to find at least an hour a day, six days a week for going to the gym.

When I interviewed Ulrich Demplfe, the founder of CAROL Bike, a workout bike that offers the same benefits of a 45 minutes cardio workout in just five minutes, he told me that the biggest barrier that prevents people from exercising is time. I couldn't agree more, and the majority of my clients, the busy executives, entrepreneurs, first responders, etc., don't have the time. Ulrich wanted to do something about that so he created the CAROL Bike. It uses AI (Artificial Intelligence) technology to match your resistance correctly.

The CAROL Bike's technology leans on the science of Reduced Exertion High-Intensity Training (REHIT) workouts. REHIT triggers your body's "fight or flight response," causing it to burn the sugar stored in your muscles as fuel. Like High-Intensity Interval Training (HIIT), REHIT workouts alternate short bursts of intense exercise with recovery periods. The difference is that REHIT workouts involve fewer, shorter bursts performed at maximum intensity. Although there are several REHIT protocols to choose from, its most popular protocol is the 5-10 minute workout that consists of a warm-up, two 20-second bursts of all-out work with a recovery period in between, and a cooldown. For example, a REHIT workout on the CAROL Bike may consist of a 2-minute warm-up, a 20-second all-out sprint, a 3-minute recovery, a 20-second all-out sprint, and a 3-minute cooldown.

Beyond the savings in time, these REHIT workouts are also tremendously beneficial for your metabolic health. Studies have shown that when participants performed REHIT workouts just three times a week for eight weeks, their metabolic measures improved across the board. This included weight loss, a drop in type-2 diabetes by 62%, and an increase in VO2 Max (a measure of how well your body can transport oxygen) by about 12%.[25]

I wanted to share this with you because there are technologies and workout principles we can utilize to save time and still be healthy. And I'm not just making this up. There's plenty of science, as you can see, to back up what I'm saying. It's all about working out smarter, not necessarily harder.

But Joel, I'm Injured, I Hate Lifting Weights, I'm Not Ready for High-Intensity Workouts....

No problem! Although I think high-intensity and variable resistance training are the best options when it comes to body transformation and overall weight loss, there are some other

---

25 Tom F. Cuddy, Joyce S. Ramos, and Lance C. Dalleck, "Reduced Exertion High-Intensity Interval Training is More Effective at Improving Cardiorespiratory Fitness and Cardiometabolic Health than Traditional Moderate-Intensity Continuous Training," *International Journal of Environmental Research and Public Health 16,* no. 3 (February 2019): 483, https://doi.org/10.3390/ijerph16030483.

things busy professionals should consider when trying to lose weight long-term.

1. Exercise Snacking: This is a concept I stress to all of my clients. It can be done by anyone at any fitness level, but it is especially beneficial for people who are *not* yet ready for high-intensity training. With Exercise Snacking, you work out for 30 minutes per day, but you break up your workout into three, 10-minute sessions that are spread out throughout the day. Within those 10-minute sessions, you warm up and then work out at an intensity that fits your fitness level. This may be light or moderate intensity to begin with, and then you can build up from there. You then end that 10-minute session with a cool down.

These short bouts of exercise spread across the day have received attention as a time-efficient exercise strategy that has more positive effects on your metabolism than a single, 30-minute workout. In one study, Francois et al. [15] identified that Exercise Snacking before each meal, consisting of six discrete minutes of exercise separated by one minute of rest, improved glycemic control the following day in middle-aged adults with impaired glucose handling. In another study, Jenkins et al. [16] reported improvements in cardiorespiratory fitness in healthy inactive adults performing three sets of maximum effort 60-step stair climbs a day, three times a week, for six weeks. The improvement in exercise tolerance included an increase in maximum power output during a VO2 peak test on a cycle ergometer [16].

This suggests that an Exercise Snacking model may have the potential to improve function beyond just cardiovascular fitness.[26]

2. Greasing the Groove: According to Pavel Tsatsouline, former Soviet special forces instructor and the father of the kettlebell in the West, "Strength is a Skill." And, like any skill, it's one you've got to work at consistently. One of the ways to build the skill of strength is through Pavel's concept of "greasing the groove." The idea here is to actually build on a specific skill through consistent practice. For example, if you wanted to get better at doing pull-ups, break up your day so that every hour you can do five pull-ups. By the end of the day, you will have done around 50 pull-ups. Now picture trying to do those 50 pull-ups during one session at the gym. In that case, it would take a long time, it would place a lot of wear and tear on your body, it would increase your risk for injury, and it would be exhausting. But, by spreading out those 50 pull-ups throughout the day and simply building them into your routine, you not only get better at that specific skill, but you also create a practice of regular movement that eliminates the sedentary lifestyle that is crushing a vast amount of Americans.

3.NEAT: More and more studies are showing that things like Non-Exercise Activity Thermogenesis (NEAT), which is

---

26 Oliver J. Perkin, Polly M. McGuigan, and Keith A. Stokes, "Exercise Snacking to Improve Muscle Function in Healthy Older Adults: A Pilot Study," *Journal of Aging Research* (October 2019): 7516939, https://doi.org/10.1155/2019/7516939.

essentially energy expenditure associated with spontaneous movements such as fidgeting while you're sitting at your desk, can help combat obesity when they are done regularly. These somewhat unplanned and unstructured low-level physical activities, including walking to work, typing, performing yard work, undertaking agricultural tasks, fidgeting, etc., are associated with energy expenditure in excess of the resting metabolic rate (RMR).

Studying the potential for converting these kinds of daily energy expenditures into a form of exercise is of great interest because most obese individuals have no exercise activity-related thermogenesis (EAT). Their physical activity-related energy expenditure (PEE) is comprised almost entirely of NEAT. Consequently, NEAT represents the main variable component of daily total energy expenditure (TEE). This varies considerably, both within and among individuals, but it does have the potential to stimulate greater energy expenditure over time for individuals who choose to have a higher adherence rate with turning their NEAT activities into more exercise-like activities.

In fact, as I'm writing this book in November of 2022, an article was published in *The National Library of Medicine* about a study showing that doing calf raises while sitting down can actually help with metabolic health and "improved systemic VLDL-triglyceride and glucose homeostasis by a large magnitude, e.g., 52% less postprandial glucose excursion (~50 mg/dL less between ~1 and 2 h) with 60% less hyperinsulinemia.[27]

Granted, the participants in this study were doing these calf raises for hours to create this effect. Nonetheless, it's exciting to see how simple, isolated contractions from such a small muscle group can have such downstream effects on metabolic health.

4. **Post-Prandial Walking:** This is a fancy term for a simple activity - taking a walk after you eat a meal. There is a belief that walking just after a meal causes fatigue, stomach ache, and discomfort so people avoid walking after eating a meal. However, studies have shown that participants had no such negative reactions. Instead, it was found that walking just after a meal was more effective for weight loss than waiting one hour after eating before walking. For people who do not experience abdominal pain, fatigue, or other discomforts when walking just after a meal, walking at a brisk speed for 30 minutes as soon as possible just after lunch and dinner lead to more weight loss than walking for 30 minutes beginning one hour after a meal had been consumed.

This research into post-prandial walking was confirmed for me when I interviewed Josh Clemente, the founder of Levels

---

27 Marc T. Hamilton, Deborah G. Hamilton, and Theodore W. Zderic, "A potent physiological method to magnify and sustain soleus oxidative metabolism improves glucose and lipid regulation," *iScience 25,* no. 9 (August 2022): 104869, https://doi.org/10.1016/j.isci.2022.104869.

Health, an app that provides real-time feedback on how your diet and lifestyle choices impact your metabolic health through biosensors like continuous glucose monitors. He told me that the most effective thing he's seen in all his research and data collecting for blunting a spike in your glucose (which, over time, has been associated with metabolic disorders such as obesity), is the post-prandial walk.

Taken together, these exercise ideas and strategies, from high-intensity and variable resistance training to post-prandial walking and everything in between, destroy the belief that we need to be in the gym six days a week for an hour daily to make a dent in weight loss.

Moreover, this variety of exercise options highlights an important fact. You should constantly vary your exercise routine for the best long-term results. Contracting and elongating your muscles hundreds or thousands of times during exercise forces them to deplete the fuel in their internal storage tanks, including glycogen and triglycerides (the storage form of fatty acids). All forms of exercise burn both glucose and fatty acids simultaneously, and your muscles always oxidize multiple fuels simultaneously. Shorter workouts with higher intensity tend to burn more glucose as fuel, whereas longer workouts with lower intensity use up those fatty acids as fuel. For these reasons, having a movement practice that covers multiple fitness domains will maximize your chances of improving insulin sensitivity and long-term metabolic health.

I am Living Proof…

Since the birth of my first son eight and half years ago, my days of working out in the gym for 60 minutes, five days a week were over. Before he was born, I was doing Crossfit and Brazilian jiu-jitsu. I remember my wife asking me, "Joel, you think you'll keep up these things when the baby is born?" I told her, "Absolutely. Do you know who I am?" I've always been goal-oriented, and whatever I put my mind to, I can achieve…."

Well, I was wrong. My wife stopped working to care of our newborn, and I had to work overtime to make up for those lost wages. Also, not sure if you know this, but having kids is hard work (Lol)! At the time, I felt like I couldn't be present and be a good dad to my newborn and maintain that workout schedule and work extra hours at work. And, by the time my second son was born three years later, I had even less time. I had to figure out a way to be physically active with little to no time because I craved physical activity since it had been a part of me for so long.

So, how did I personally optimize my workouts for the little time I had? My methods have evolved and changed over time. I've also adopted and added new technologies to my fitness regimen since my sons were born. For instance, I recently added the CAROL Bike to my exercise arsenal. But, here's a list of things that I prioritized at the beginning of this journey that still hold true today:

1. **Daily Movement Practice:** I do at least 20 minutes a day of non-high-intensity exercise every day. It can be as simple as walking, stretching, or mobility work.

2. **Consistency:** I don't miss many days of my movement practice. Over the last eight and a half years, I've maintained some form of movement practice for 5-6 days a week, every week.

3. **Outdoor Workouts:** I exercise outside regularly, even when it's cold and snowing. Outside workouts serve a few purposes. First, they help to optimize your Vitamin D levels when you absorb sunlight through your skin. This is important because research has shown over and over that high vitamin D levels correlate with better immunity and overall longevity. Second, when conditions permit, you can combine your outdoor exercise with a practice that is known as 'grounding.' The purpose of grounding is to have direct physical contact with the vast supply of electrons on the surface of the Earth. Modern lifestyle separates humans from such contact. The research suggests that this disconnect may be a major contributor to physiological dysfunction and unwellness. Reconnection with the Earth's electrons has been found to promote intriguing physiological changes and subjective reports of well-being.[28] In order to practice

---

28 James L Oschman, Gaétan Chevalier, and Richard Brown, "The effects of grounding (earthing) on inflammation, the immune response, wound healing, and prevention and treatment of chronic inflammatory and autoimmune diseases," *Journal of Inflammation Research,* no. 8 (March 2015): 83–96, https://doi.org/10.2147/JIR.S69656.

grounding, simply remove your socks and shoes and allow your bare feet to make contact with the earth for your next outdoor workout

4. **X3 Bar:** I invested early in this product when it first came out. Dr. John Jaquish, the inventor, had studied bone density and osteoporosis for years and realized that, using the principle of variable resistance, he could trigger muscles to grow three times greater (hence the name X3). This led Dr. Jaquish to create a portable platform that uses latex bands (resistance bands) to create a variable resistance training system that can fit in everyone's home. The product might seem gimmicky and fake at first glance, but I've used it for the last eight and half years to maintain my muscle mass, burn body fat, and keep my high-intensity workouts to 10 minutes daily.

By combining these principles and technologies, I have been able to maintain a great physical shape that makes me comfortable in my own body and fills me with the energy I need to balance my many endeavors with my most important job - being a husband and father. After many years of devoting lots of time and energy to going to the gym, I would not have believed that this was possible until I had to make the change in my exercise lifestyle and saw the results for myself. So, when I tell you it's possible to only work out 10, 20, or 30 minutes every day and still maintain a physique that you and your family can be proud of, I'm not lying.

ACTION STEPS

1. **Ignite Your Mitochondria!:** If it is hard to get motivated to exercise or if making time for exercise feels overwhelming, remember that your energy, brain functioning, and hormonal balance all improve with exercise because exercise improves your mitochondria. So, get those "power plants" working and start to feel better in every way.

2. **Stop Doing Cardio, and Start Doing Resistance Training:** Swap out cortisol for growth hormone and testosterone by putting your time and energy into high-intensity and variable resistance training. You can use weights, some type of latex bands, or even attach bands to your weights while doing resistance training. The goal is to work to the point of full fatigue so that your body will start burning fat and building muscle.

3. **Move as Often as Possible:** You should supplement your workouts with movement throughout the day. This can be in the form of Exercise Snacking, Greasing the Groove, NEAT movements, Post-Prandial Walks, etc. But, no matter where you may be on your exercise and fitness journey, just find a way to get moving and keep moving.

4. **Invest in Exercise Technology:** Necessity is the Mother of Invention, and people have needed to find ways to workout that are effective while not being time-consuming and that can be done in the comfort of your own home rather than at the gym. We get to benefit from the inventions that arose from those needs. If possible, invest in an X3

Bar (Use code JOEL at checkout) and/or in a CAROL Bike (Use Code JOELEVAN at checkout).

Scan the QR code below to get a list of my top exercise gear, hacks, and favorite workouts.

Chapter 7

Sleep/Recovery

Sleeping five to six hours was associated with a more than 50% increased risk of weight gain. The more sleep deprivation, the more weight gain.

-Dr. James Fung

One of my mentors, multi-millionaire and ultra-successful sports marketer and philanthropist, David Meltzer, mentioned to me that he has a sleep coach. When I heard him say this, I couldn't believe it. Why would anyone pay for a sleep coach? What do they tell you to do? Go to bed earlier? Fluff your pillows? I mean, really. But then I took a step back and thought, "Dave already has a nutrition coach, he already has a trainer, and he's trying to optimize everything in his life. The only thing missing was sleep." This guy is winning in life, but he realized that sleep was one area where he could improve. He also realized that if could sleep better, then the other areas of his life could improve even more. We may not all be multi-millionaires who can invest in sleep coaches; however, the point is this: if an enormously successful man like Dave Meltzer feels the need to invest in a sleep coach, then why aren't the rest of us at least paying a little more attention to our sleep?

Of course, we all know how important sleep is for our health and wellness. We may even love sleep and look forward to sleeping. Yet, we do not prioritize our sleep. One reason for this disconnect is that we are living a "there are not enough hours in the day" lifestyle in which proper sleep takes a back seat to everything else that we need to cram into our days. Another reason for this disconnect is that we've gotten used to getting by without adhering to the well-known standard of sleeping eight hours per night. I've even seen many clients dial in most of their eating habits and exercise but overlook and scoff at sleep when I mention it. If you're not sleeping enough, most likely stress is still high. When stress is high, your stress hormone, cortisol is high. As we've learned already, chronically high levels of cortisol can tell your body to hold on to bodyfat.

Even if you feel like you are managing "just fine" on less sleep, I promise you that it is affecting you in negative ways. In fact, it is actually affecting you right down to your hormones, and it is affecting your ability to lose weight. Knowing this, I try to emphasize the need for proper sleep with my clients because poor sleep habits can derail all your efforts to be as healthy as possible. You have come this far in this book, and you may have started taking the recommended steps in your holistic weight loss journey - do not let poor sleep habits be your kryptonite.

Blue Light Exposure

Nature is very smart. Our bodies and brains are linked to the cycles of the sun. Blue light is a spectrum of light that is naturally found in our sun during the day. It tells our bodies, "It's time to wake up; it's time to go." Then, when the sun sets, you see more of the purple and red spectrum of light from the sun. This is not by accident. When these spectrums hit our eyes, it tells our brains, "It's time to down-regulate and prepare for sleep." Unfortunately, we don't live this way in our modern society.

Instead, we have disrupted this natural sleep/wake cycle by flooding our homes and our lives with artificially created blue light. All of our electronics and the LED light bulbs in our homes emit blue light waves. To make matters worse, most of us stay on our electronics until the last minute before our heads hit our pillows.

Maybe you have heard this before, and you know that blue light is "bad" for your sleep and that you should try to minimize your blue light exposure before bed. But, how "bad" is "bad," and what does "bad" for your sleep really mean?

Well, several studies have shown that blue light isn't just bad for our sleep, it is actually detrimental to our overall well-being.

This extends well beyond feeling less energized after a bad night's sleep. Artificial blue light exposure is now understood to be a contributor to insulin resistance and, therefore, obesity.

One study looking at blue light's effects on insulin and obesity found the following:

The study showed that blue-enriched light exposure acutely altered metabolic function in the morning and the evening compared to dim light. While morning and evening blue-enriched light exposure both resulted in higher insulin resistance, evening blue-enriched light led to higher peak glucose. This suggests a greater inability of insulin to adequately compensate for the increase in glucose in the evening.[29]

Melatonin

Blue light also affects other hormones, such as melatonin. Melatonin is a key hormone and antioxidant in our body. It facilitates cell repair and quells inflammation. It also helps us fall asleep. Mariana Figuero, PhD, of the Lighting Research Center at Rensselaer Polytechnic Institute in Troy, New York, and her team showed that just two hours of computer

---

29   Ivy N. Cheung, Phyllis C. Zee, Dov Shalman, Roneil G. Malkani, Joseph Kang, and Kathryn J. Reid, "Morning and Evening Blue-Enriched Light Exposure Alters Metabolic Function in Normal Weight Adults," *PLoS One 11,* no. 5 (May 2016): e0155601, https://doi.org/10.1371/journal.pone.0155601.

screen time before bed was enough to significantly suppress people's nighttime release of melatonin. When your melatonin secretion is thrown off, it takes you longer to fall asleep, and you wake up feeling less restful. A recent Harvard Study comparing different colored light waves showed, "The blue light suppressed melatonin for about twice as long as the green light and shifted circadian rhythms by twice as much (3 hours vs. 1.5 hours)."[30]

Moreover, studies are showing that melatonin plays an important role in keeping other hormones in balance. There are several good studies showing that melatonin supplementation has both a positive effect on weight loss as well as an ability to rebalance hormonal imbalances. One study for example, showed "that melatonin supplementation had a beneficial effect on the secretion of leptin, adiponectin and on the level of glucose, cholesterol (LDL) and triglycerides, particularly in animals with induced obesity."[31] I've talked already about the importance of glucose metabolism and insulin. Well, in regards to insulin resistance, "patients with obesity taking melatonin for 12 weeks show a pronounced decrease in

---

30 "Blue light has a dark side," Harvard Health Publishing, Harvard Medical School, July 7, 2020, https://www.health.harvard.edu/staying-healthy/blue-light-has-a-dark-side.

31 Ewa Walecka-Kapica et al., "The effect of melatonin supplementation on the quality of sleep and weight status in postmenopausal women," *Menopause Review Przeglad Menopauzalny 13,* no. 6 (December 2014): 334–338, https://doi.org/10.5114/pm.2014.47986.

the insulin resistance (IR) index.[32] More and more men and women are complaining about their hormones being off. We're seeing an uptick in women needing IVF to have children and men needing testosterone replacement therapy (TRT) at an earlier age. What if optimizing your sleep could reverse a lot of these issues?

Cortisol

In addition, we know from multiple studies that there is a connection between our gut and our brain and that proper sleep makes our guts happier. Lack of sleep increases cortisol and other stress hormones, putting your body into a state of fight or flight. When the nervous system is revved up, cortisol can trigger "bad bacteria" to fester throughout the microbiome. Insufficient sleep could alter your microbiome, throw off the absorption of food nutrients, and cause gastrointestinal problems.

This overproduction of cortisol doesn't just lead to digestion problems, it also hinders your ability to lose weight. A study was conducted on overweight men and women. One group was sleep deprived, the other was not, and they both went on a strict, low-calorie diet for two weeks. Weight loss occurred in both groups; however, in the sleep-deprived group, more than

---

32 Hang Sun, Xingchun Wang, Jiaqi Chen, Aaron M. Gusdon, Kexiu Song, Liang Li, and Shen Qu, "Melatonin treatment improves insulin resistance and pigmentation in obese patients with acanthosis nigricans," *International Journal of Endocrinology* (2018): 2304746, https://doi.org/10.1155/2018/2304746.

70% of the pounds lost came from lean body mass muscle, not fat. When you lack sleep, cortisol is increased, and the body is reluctant to give up fat.

Sleep and Appetite

Dr. Matthew Walker, sleep expert and author of *Why We Sleep: Unlocking the Power of Sleep and Dreams*, discovered that brain activity is altered when we do not get a full night of sleep. The functioning of the pre-frontal cortex, the part of our brain that is involved in executive functioning and making good judgments and controlled decisions, is impaired by lack of sleep. In contrast, the functioning of the limbic system, the parts of our brain that are involved with primal functioning and making decisions based on emotion and arousal, is more activated by a lack of sleep. Studies show that sleep-deprived people are more stimulated when shown images of food.

Beyond impacting your ability to make good choices, including good food choices, insufficient sleep also directly impairs your ability to regulate your appetite. Dr. Eve Van Cauter, at the University of Chicago, has conducted massive amounts of study and research on the link between sleep and appetite. In the course of her research, she found that more than one-third of individuals in industrialized societies sleep less than five to six hours a night during the week. She also found that disrupted sleep can alter your leptin and ghrelin levels, which are hormones that help regulate appetite.

In one of Dr. Van Cauter's studies, a group of individuals who slept eight and half hours for five days straight was compared to a second group who only slept four to five hours a night for five days straight. Both groups were given the same amount and type of food. They also did the same amount of physical activity. Each day, the sense of hunger and food intake were monitored in both groups, and their blood was checked for circulating levels of leptin and ghrelin. Dr. Van Cauter found that individuals were "far more ravenous when sleeping four to five hours a night."[33] Interestingly, a strong rise in hunger and increased reported appetite occurred quickly. It happened within the second day for those study participants who were sleeping only four to five hours a night.

Dr. Van Cauter conducted a second study to see if "feeling hungry" led to more eating when sleeping less. Van Cauter organized two groups: one group that slept eight and a half hours a night for four nights with free access to food and a second group that slept four and a half hours a night for four nights with free access to food. The group that was only sleeping four and a half hours a night ate, on average, 300 more calories a day than the group sleeping eight and a half hours a night. This amounted to well over 1,000 calories before the end of the experiment. In other experiments where the sleep-deprived group slept five to six hours a night, which is a common amount of sleep for many Americans, the findings were similar. Scale these numbers up to a working year, and

---

33 Matthew Walker, *Why We Sleep: Unlocking the Power of Sleep and Dreams* (New York, NY: Scribner, 2018), 172.

most people will have consumed more than 70,000 extra calories, leading to 10-15 pounds of weight gain a year.

In other research, Dr. Van Cauter added an experiment to the final day of a sleep/appetite study. For this experiment, both groups of people, the well-rested and the sleep-deprived, were given free access to a buffet with an assortment of foods and a dessert snack bar. Despite eating almost 2,000 calories during the buffet lunch, sleep-deprived participants dove into the snack bar. They consumed an additional 330 calories of snack foods compared to the study participants who were fully rested. This led Dr. Van Cauter to observe that sleep-deprived participants sought out heavy-hitting carbohydrate-rich foods, salty snacks, and sugary sweets more often and in greater quantities than their fully rested counterparts. This all increased by 30-40% when sleep was further reduced by several hours a night.

My Sleep & Weight Loss

As you may have guessed by now, I like to confirm my research by comparing it to my own lived experiences. This helps me to make better choices for myself and for my clients. To this end, I recently was wearing a continuous glucose monitor (CGM) to track my glucose levels. As we now know, controlling and balancing our glucose levels is important for long-term health and longevity. I typically wake up at 4:00 am and get my day started, and I typically try to get to bed before 10:00 pm. That's about six hours of sleep in total. When I woke up one morning,

I checked my CGM, and it showed that my real-time blood glucose levels were 120. This was not optimal at all. I tell all my clients that when they wake up, having a fasting glucose of 100 or below is optimal. Mainstream Western doctors consider 95 to be the optimal fasting glucose. However, many experts in my cohort and other functional medicine doctors believe that a healthy fasting glucose is around 85.

So, when I woke up with a score of 120, you can imagine I was a little flummoxed. I remembered what I had eaten the night before, and the foods weren't terrible. I also had done a minimum of 12 hours of fasting. So what was the issue? Well, I recalled that I had stayed up later than I normally do and that I was on the computer, surrounded by blue light. The following night, I made sure I avoided blue light right before bed, I went to bed early at 9:00 pm, and I slept until 5:00 am. When I awoke the following morning after my eight hours of sleep, my glucose reading was exactly 85. Although there are several other variables, my meals and types of food overall had stayed the same that second night. The only thing that changed was my nighttime routine and more sleep. For me, this is the proof, backed by the research, that good quality sleep can truly improve your metabolic health.

The 4-Hour Critical Window: 10:00 pm – 2:00 am

When you are creating your new sleep habits, it is important to keep in mind how our bodies work and what is happening to our bodies during sleep. In a nutshell, sleep is our body's way of replenishing all that it has used up during our waking hours. Sleep is recovery. In his book *Sleep Smarter: 21 Essential Strategies to Sleep Your Way to a Better Body, Better Health and Bigger Success,* Shawn Stevenson outlines research suggesting "human beings get the most beneficial hormonal secretions and recovery by sleeping during the hours of 10:00 pm to 2:00 am."[34] In addition, our stress glands (adrenals) rest and recharge the most between 11:00 pm and 1:00 am, and melatonin production is highest between 10:00 pm to 2:00 am. Based on these factors, I always recommend that my clients aim to be asleep for this 4-hour critical window (*Note*: I understand that this may be impossible for people, like first responders, who work night shifts. But, I still encourage them to focus on the quality and quantity of their sleep).

There is No Downside to More Sleep

Above all, if you are putting effort into improving your sleep habits and things seem hard at first, keep the big picture in mind. Know that sleeping more does not "take away" the time you need to get things done. Instead, it only makes you more efficient and productive because more sleep improves your executive functioning. You can get more done in less time when you aren't struggling with decision-making. Furthermore, when sleeping more helps regulate your hormones and your appetite, you will lose weight and gain energy. This too will

---

34 Shawn Stevenson, *Sleep Smarter: 21 Essential Strategies to Sleep Your Way to a Better Body, Better Health, and Bigger Success* (Houston, TX: Audible Studios, 2016).

improve your ability to accomplish more in less time. Plus, by following my advice about diet and exercise, you have streamlined both of these daily necessities and given yourself more time in your day. Why not put that time toward sleep? Finally, many people assume you'll burn more calories when you're awake. However, this is not true. Instead, sleep is "an intensely metabolically active state for brain and body alike." Even if you stayed up 24 hours straight, you'd only burn an extra 147 calories compared to the calories you'd burn while sleeping a full eight hours. Let good sleep ignite your metabolism and propel you on your weight loss journey.

Sleep Hygiene

Now you might be saying, "All right, Joel, I believe you. I know I need to sleep more. But I'm so used to sleeping less than eight hours a night that I always wake up after just five or six hours. How do I make myself sleep more? First, remember what I told you in Chapter 3, the brain likes habits. Your sleep pattern is a habit. Second, remember the principles I taught you about habit breaking and habit building. You need to break your bad sleep habits and build good sleep habits. The way to do so is by improving your sleep hygiene. Sleep hygiene is your own individual program for sleep. Just like you have maintain your personal hygiene by taking showers daily and brushing your teeth two times a day, we need stop prioritizing sleep the same way. How do you get good at sleep? As silly as it sounds, you create a plan for it. For my own personal plan, I know that by 8 pm every night, I stop working and I shut out bluelight completely from my environment. Below, I'll list some tactical things you can do that have worked for the majority of my clients and helped shift their sleeping habits.

ACTION STEPS

1. Keep **a Sleep Journal**: Evaluate your sleep and notice if you're not prioritizing it. Keep track of when you go to sleep and wake up, what you were doing before you went to bed, what activities and routines help and hurt your ability to fall asleep and stay asleep, etc.

2. **Create a Bedtime Routine**: Bedtime routines aren't just for children. Think about how and why they do work for children and apply this to your own quest for better sleep. The key to good sleep is a consistent schedule around going to bed and waking up. Studies back this up, and I have seen the same from tracking my sleep for over four years with an Oura ring.

3. **Invest in Your Sleep:** My favorite bio hacks for sleep are black-out curtains for creating a pitch-dark environment, keeping the bedroom at 68 degrees or cooler, and wearing blue-light-blocking glasses at least 2 hours before bed. I like TrueDark red glasses, but there are several good companies.

4. **Hot Showers:** Hot showers or baths have worked for many people as they help rapidly cool the internal temperature of the body upon exiting. Having a cool internal temperature

as been shown to be extremely beneficial for reaching deep sleep levels quicker and longer. Check out my podcast with Tara Youngblood, the founder of SleepMe and ChilliSleep to learn more (Episode #189).

5. **Remove BlueLight Two Hours Before Bed:** At least two hours before you're planning to put your head on the pillow, began to remove blue light from your environment. You can do this by investing in blue blocking glasses like I've already mentioned, which is probably the easiest for most people. This way, they can still enjoy all the delights of modern technology, but simply block it out with a pair of glasses. You could also remove the majority of blue lights in your home and replace them with blue light blocking bulbs.

6. **Targeted Supplementation:** I think everyone can benefit from taking a magnesium supplement as the majority of Americans are deficient in magnesium. Magnesium is magical mineral that is known to having calming and relaxing effects on the body. The best forms of magnesium for body relaxation and sleep would be magnesium citrate and glycinate. You could also try experimenting with magnesium threonate, which directly effects the neurons in the brain. See my podcast also with Dr. Barb Woegerer, an expert in magnesium and all the different forms (Episode #190).

The second supplement backed by a ton of research would be melatonin. I like a liquid form of melatonin so I can titrate the doses even 0.5-1.5 mg just to help nudge clients to sleep. The liquid version seems to also help them feel less groggy even at higher doses.

I've also used essential oils on my kids and have received a lot of feedback from our community that oils such as doTerra's Serenity, Balance, Adaptiv, Roman Chamomile, and Lavendar have helped restore people's sleep and lower their anxiety.

7. **Breathwork:** Practice meditation or breathwork prior to bed. Something as simple as box breathing: breathing in for four seconds, holding for four seconds, breathing for four seconds, and holding for four seconds. Do this for 10 minutes, and you will create a relaxed state one that is known as coherence. I like to think of coherence as being aligned with your heart and body.

8. **Mouth-Breathing:** Most people are mouth breathers, which leads to snoring and interrupted sleep. I personally use MyoTape, which is a brand of mouth tape that keeps my mouth from opening during the night, forcing me to breath in through my nose, the way mother nature created us.

9. **Unplug Your Wifi**: Listen, whether you believe it or not we are being bombarded by all types of radio waves and electromagnetic frequencies (EMF's) that are harmful to our system. Many people are sensitive to EMF's and by just removing them from their lifestyle or limiting their exposure (the same way you'd remove a certain food from your body), they've seen positive results. Personally, I do

this every night and make sure if my phone is near me at night, it's on airplane mode. I've also invested in technology like Somavedic and LeelaQ Tech, which create devices that help harmonize your environment from the negative EMF's. They can't block them completely, but they can at least neutralize the negative frequency in a way that's harmonious for your environment.

10. **Binaural Beats:** Binaural beat therapy is an emerging form of sound wave therapy. It makes use of the fact that the right and left ear each receive a slightly different frequency tone, yet the brain perceives these as a single tone. For example, if the left ear registers a tone at 200 Hz and the right ear registers one at 210 Hz, the binaural beat is 10 Hz — the difference between the two frequencies. The idea is to play binaural beats and music in your ears to entrain the brain into a certain frequency or state such as gamma (higher consciousness), delta (slow wave/deep sleep), theta (meditation/REM sleep), and alpha (focused/relaxation). There are several free and paid apps out there that deliver this technology. One popular app is called Brain.fm which I've used for years and like. The problem with binaural beats according to the experts, is that over time, the brain will learn the patterns of the beats, and it will no longer be effective.

A couple technologies I use regularly that have claimed to solve that problem are NuCalm and BrainTap. Nucalm creates binaural beats that are delivered through an app just like many of the free apps out there. The difference is that there sound files are almost 700 megabytes. The tracks are made in a way that are so intricate, the brain can never pickup on the pattern no matter how many times you listen to it. One of NuCalm's most popular tracks is played for only 20 minutes, and is said to be the equivalent of two hours of deep sleep. I've personally seen a lot of success in my sleep, rest, and recovery using this app.

BrainTap is another one that I've mentioned earlier in the book. They use light and sound (binaural beats) via a headset to entrain the brain as well. BrainTap understands the downfall of binaural beats, which is why when I interviewed the founder, Dr. Patrick Porter, he said he's created over 1,000 tracks on the app to make it impossible for the brain to learn the patterns. I've gotten huge success with this technology as well and have seen my HRV score (a measure of of rest/recovery) skyrocket in the morning, just from listening to a sleep track the night before (this was highly noticeable as I regularly track my sleep, and I got an enormous increase in HRV the following morning, which was abnormal for me).

Scan the QR code below to get a list of my top sleep & recovery resources.

Chapter 8

Prioritize & Execute

Without struggle, there is no progress. Embrace the struggle, and remember that a setback, is a setup for a comeback.

-Dr. Eric Thomas

You have all the tools. You know what it takes to lose weight and feel healthier, more energized, and more comfortable in your own body. You know all the practices, the nutrition, the exercise program, and the hacks. Now it comes down to one thing - consistency.

I remember doing a weekly check-in with one of my clients after he'd already lost 25 pounds, and he wanted to lose an additional 10 pounds. We looked at any of the gaps that needed to be tightened up to get him to those last 10 pounds, and we discovered that he needed more physical movement and better sleep.

After his first week of implementing the new game plan, he said he lost two more pounds. But, after just one day of eating a flex meal, he gained the two pounds back. He sounded defeated and disappointed. He said, "Joel, after all the work I put in, it seems like I should have lost more…" I laughed and reminded him, "Yes, it's true, but you've only been doing this new game plan for one week."

Don't Make This Mistake

Most of us are looking for the next big thing or the magic pill that will solve all of our problems. We want a quick, easy fix, immediate gratification, and instant results. We want to read a book like this then, when we are excited and feeling motivated, we want to implement the strategies and suggestions. Yet, almost as soon as we get started, we also want to see results. This is the biggest mistake I see people make after going through a coaching program or reading a book like this one. You read it once, make some changes, and then think, "I've got it."

But, remember my client's story. He was disappointed and frustrated after only one week of implementing our new plan. When we are narrow-focused, when we want instant results, when we think "I've got it," then it's easy to get disgruntled when our progress is slow or we have setbacks. Weight loss, and, for that matter, any other worthy life goal, is a long-haul journey. We need to settle in for the ride.

So, how do you prepare yourself to stay the course and succeed through the twists and turns and ups and downs of this journey? The answer comes back full circle to the beginning of this book. You must have the proper perspective and a consistent mindset practice in order to achieve long-term success.

That's why I put mindset at the forefront of this weight loss program. Without that rock-solid foundation, the likelihood of you following through and staying consistent with any part of this program will be slim-to-none.

Therefore, it is imperative to understand that mindset is not something you get overnight. Mindset is an everyday job that we all have to work at consistently. Don't ever think you've got it. You can't just sit back and think your success is on auto-pilot. Old beliefs will trigger you and come up. The mind naturally will default to these old beliefs because they're ingrained in the subconscious. It's your job to continually detach and make mindset a daily practice.

Remember, though, your mindset practice is not an additional chore or burden in your life. Instead, it is about removing interference from your life. There's nothing you need to add to what you're doing. You actually need to subtract what's getting in your way from being the highest version of yourself. Many of us are not living the highest version of ourselves. We aren't aligned with our truth. We are living fake lives made up of someone else's beliefs, pretending to be living a life we enjoy. That's why every new diet fad or exercise program will only last for a little bit and will never stick long-term. You never looked under the hood and did some of the deep work. Until you work on your mind and establish the discipline that emphasizes health as a priority, you'll always be chasing quick fixes and doing patchwork on your body and mind.

Anytime a client has a breakdown or stumbles in their diet, I always ask, "How's the mindset work going?" Ten out of ten times, they tell me, "I stopped doing it," or "I kind of forgot…I missed a few days…" Always.

I'm telling you, you don't have a diet problem. You don't have an exercise problem. You have a mindset problem.

Condition Yellow

Okay, Joel. I get it. But, how do I evolve and keep working on developing my mindset? First, you need to develop your mindset awareness. To do so, it helps to have a working knowledge of Jeff Cooper's "Color Codes of Awareness." Cooper was a United States Marine who developed a system whereby the different levels of human awareness were matched to a specific color. Although his Color Code system is decades old, it is still used in self-defense instruction and in military and first responder training because it is effective and simple. In this system, Condition White means that you have no awareness of what is happening around you, Condition Yellow means that you are relaxed but are aware of your surroundings and paying attention, Condition Orange means that you have identified something of interest that may or may not prove to be a threat, and Condition Red means that you must be ready to defend yourself because you have an immediate threat.

In terms of your weight loss mindset, which is, of course, synonymous with your goal-achieving mindset, Condition White is the easiest level of awareness to understand. Just like you know that you should not walk through a dark alley with your headphones in, your face in your phone, and your thoughts a million miles away, you understand that a complete lack of awareness about your goals only invites trouble. You cannot possibly succeed in your weight loss journey if you never think about your habits, your goals, your diet, your exercise, and so on.

Condition Red, though more complex than Condition White, might be the next easiest level of awareness to understand. For first responders and the military, having a Condition Red level awareness is sometimes a necessary part of the job. Although you may not be a first responder or in the military, you probably have some experience with Condition Red - especially during the Covid Pandemic. Prior to the Pandemic, we went about our business and simply sat on planes, trains and buses, ate in restaurants, and went into stores. But, all of a sudden, we were told to be hypervigilant about the strangers around us because they could be potential threats to our health. From this experience, you can see that Condition Red is a place of such stress and strain that it cannot and should not be a permanent state of awareness.

In terms of your weight loss journey, this means two things for your mindset. First, you may read a book like this and start to look at your food, exercise, habits, etc. in a whole new light. You may become hypervigilant about these things. Do not let your new knowledge overwhelm you and turn into a source of stress. Second, as I mentioned earlier in this book, studies suggest that the average person has about 12,000 to 60,000 thoughts per day, and 80% of these thoughts are negative while 95% are repetitive thoughts from the previous day. Not only are the vast majority of our thoughts negative, the majority never come true. Yet, we spend most of our time dwelling on them. Moreover, the systems we live in are programming us to live in this heightened state of worry and stress. Imagine what that's doing for your mindset and your heart-set over time. You need to examine your own thought processes and, as much as possible, cleanse your mind of this negative clutter. It weighs you down literally and figuratively. So, get excited, be enthusiastic, and look forward to making changes in your life, but do so from a positive mindset rather than from a Condition Red mindset.

This leaves Condition Yellow and Condition Orange. For the majority of your time, have a Condition Yellow level of awareness about your weight loss mindset. You are aware, but you are not stressed. Then, when situations arise where you find that you are slipping in your mindset, you raise your awareness to a Condition Orange. For instance, you may go on vacation and pay less attention to your diet and exercise. It happens. That is fine. But, if you return from vacation and stay lax about your habits then it is time to heighten your mindset to a Condition Orange where you recognize that threats to your well-being could be lurking around the corner so you do the work to get yourself back on track toward meeting your goals.

Discipline Is Only For the Special Few

If you are thinking that this mindset work will take discipline, you are right. If you are thinking that only 'special' people like celebrities and professional athletes have the discipline needed to prioritize the health and well-being of their bodies, you are wrong. The truth is that you are as worthy of having a fit and healthy body as any public figure. In fact, the most successful people I've met are not any more special than anyone else. Instead, they are regular people who made the choice to be consistent day in and day out, no matter what happens. Even when things aren't going well, they dig back into their mindset and positive self-talk, and they do it anyway. They've setup up the rituals, practices, and systems so that, no matter how they're feeling, they show up anyway. I can't stress this enough.

When I interviewed world-class trainer Steve Jordan, who has over two decades of experience in health and fitness and is the trainer for many high-end Hollywood clients, he told me that the ability to follow through is the key to success. He said that, in terms of achieving fitness goals, follow-through is probably the number one thing that is overlooked although it is the most important factor for success. It's not how you start; it's how you finish. It's the last five minutes of your exercise session. It's the last effort you give on the last set, not the first set.

Steve also said that there's no difference between a high-end Hollywood actor or actress and a "normal person." They're all human and fall to the same vices. The biggest difference, he said, is their standards. People in Hollywood typically had to do something hard to get where they are, and they want to maintain that status. Therefore, they have higher standards for themselves. If your standards are low, ask yourself why. Why don't you hold yourself to the same standards as someone you may look up to? I challenge you to constantly be raising your standards. As you evolve, your standards should evolve too.

Remember, you can have all the knowledge in the world about weight loss or any other life goal. But, it's your follow-through mindset that enables you to implement that knowledge. This fundamental truth is a cornerstone of Zander Fryer's High Impact Coaching program. Zander teaches online coaches like me to build profitable coaching businesses to six figures and beyond. I am extremely grateful that I met Zander. Not only did I learn the skills to build a profitable business, but I also strengthened my mindset and my heart-set more than ever before. Building a business and becoming a full-blown entrepreneur is not an easy task. Entrepreneurs are wired differently. As Zander says, "You have to be crazy to be an entrepreneur." Entrepreneurship is not linear, and growth is not always easy and sunshine and rainbows.

I spent over $30,000 learning from Zander and his team and being part of his Mastermind program, and I want to share some of those lessons that made the most impact on my life in terms of follow-through and execution. Following through is what separates the great from the good. How many times have you learned something, just like you've probably learned in this book or in a coaching program, but your implementation was weak? Or you implemented it for one week, but you could not sustain it for a month, or a year, or for forever. Tasks like meditation or journaling get boring, they get tedious, and they don't seem to work as much as when you first started. So you stop. The difference between you and the best in the world is they don't stop. They say, "Aha! I'm not getting much out of this. I must be on the other side of a breakthrough." And they push on and do it anyway. They prioritize consistency and a follow-through mindset.

Reflection

Perhaps you are thinking that this all sounds like it requires sound self-awareness and honest self-assessment. It definitely does. I know this first hand. I'm constantly evolving and changing as a father, as a husband and as a businessman, and I'm meeting new challenges. The other day, my wife challenged me and pointed out some of my old beliefs that I was putting on my son. It completely rocked my world. And you know what, I didn't want to hear it. I didn't want to admit that maybe those old beliefs were not serving me as a parent. Maybe those old beliefs were wrong. So, even though I have been excelling in many areas of my business and career, I realized that I always have room to learn and grow. We all do, and we all should.

I also have learned that the best way to learn and grow is to actively and consistently reflect on my successes and failures. Every month, when I was a part of Zander's Mastermind, we would get together and do a 'Deep Dive' call that would last about three hours. We'd review some core principles, get into some mindset and psychology work and then jump into some tactical things that help coaches grow their businesses.

What I noticed from these regular, monthly Deep Dives, from speaking to other Masterminds, and from having interviewed hundreds of the brightest minds in health and mastery in the world, is that successful, high-achieving people have a reflection process. Most people are really busy in their lives. They're moving a lot, and this motion creates a sense that, "I'm busy, so I must be getting work done." But, is busy being misconstrued as succeeding? Unfortunately, if busy truly isn't the same as positive forward action then no real growth is happening. Therefore, it is imperative to truly reflect on both our actions and our inactions.

Everyone should have some type of weekly review or, in the Mastermind case, a monthly review where you ask yourself, "What's the biggest thing I need to change or improve on?" To drill down this open-ended question, you also may ask yourself what is known as the **5 Power Questions for Reflection.**

The 5 Power Questions for Reflection are:

1. What do you need to stop doing?
2. What fears do you need to stop letting control you?
3. What actions do you need to do differently?
4. What beliefs do you need to let go of?
5. What people might you need to let go of?

These five questions drill into all areas of your life: your habits, the good and the bad ones; your mindset, fears, and beliefs; your tribe and the people you surround yourself with; and the actions you need to be taking. When you get down to the brass tacks like this, there's usually a concrete piece of data that will show you why something is not working.

However, the reflection process should not just focus on what you need to do better. It should also focus on what you are doing right. During your reflection, ask yourself, "What's been my biggest accomplishment? Why?" We need to constantly be celebrating ourselves. We all get so lost in the minutiae of what's not working that we lose sight of all the amazing things happening in our lives.

Without this reflection process, we have no awareness of why things are working or why they're not working. How can you improve your life if you just assume that everything is going great? For instance, if you're not losing weight and you're drinking alcohol three times a week, maybe you need to reflect on that behavior. Stop drinking alcohol and see if that contributes to better sleep, better mood, and weight loss. But, if you never reflect and decide to ask yourself that question, you will fall into the trap of routines and habits that don't serve you. This regular reflection process is really powerful for your career, health, relationships, and more. You can use it to gain some awareness of where you're at in your life and to start living the highest version of yourself.

Creating Your 2-3 Year Vision

You cannot adequately reflect on where you are in your journey unless you have a clear vision of where you want to go. This is true for weight loss, and this is true for life. In Chapter 2, we discussed vision, why it's important, and how to use a strong, clear vision to pull you closer to your dreams. We must constantly be in tune with our vision, our North Star, and where we want to go. When I spoke about vision in Chapter 2, I focused on creating a vision for your health and weight loss. But, we know that's not all there is to life. What about your income level, your business/career, and the experiences you want to have? Write out, in vivid detail, where you want to be in 2-3 years in all of these areas. List the top 3-5 things you want to accomplish in that timeframe. This is going to be your North Star. In case you ever get lost in the course of your journey, use your North Star to navigate back to the path that will take you where you want to go. Most people don't get clear on this, and that's why they're juggling ten different projects but not really accomplishing anything in any of those projects. They sound really busy, but, because they lack clarity in the top 3-5 things they really want to accomplish, they're not getting anywhere.

Prioritize & Execute

Ok, great. Having that North Star is truly invaluable. But, we really need to break the long journey down into manageable chunks. To do so, we're simply going to work backward. Look at your 2-3 year vision then chunk it down further into smaller metrics. What's your 3-6 month vision? What do you need to accomplish in the next 3-6 months that's going to eventually get you to that 2-3 year vision? Then, when you complete that leg of your journey, detail your next 3-6 month vision and so on.

To help crystalize your vision, ask yourself:

1. Does this get me to the goal?
2. Does this get me to my goal fast & efficiently?
3. What is the cost? What will I have to give up if I do this?

Remember, most of us set a goal that feels warm and fuzzy, and we get excited for a week. Then life happens. And we forget about the goal and the 2-3 year vision. Things get murky and unclear again, and we fall back into old routines and habits. The path of least resistance. We need to constantly be fighting this path of least resistance and be leaning into discomfort. We need to be constantly fighting the temptation of the next new hot thing. I'm a victim of this "shiny object syndrome" as well. I have to be doing this reflection process regularly and asking myself, "Are the actions I'm taking today moving towards my 3-5 top priority goals right now?" If the answer is no, then I need to let go of the things that are causing me to take detours on my journey.

The Rule of 3

In Jim Collin's book, *Good To Great,* he evaluated and teased out all the nuances of what made a good company a great company. One of the things he said is that great companies only have a total of 3 top priorities. He says, "If you have more than three priorities, you don't have any." Most people, he argued, need a "stop-doing list" rather than a to-do list.

Based on this concept, we're now going to break things down even smaller. We started with a mountain we want to climb, which is our 2-3 year vision. Then chunked it down to hills we want to climb, which are our 3-6 month visions. Now let's break it down even further.

What are Your:

- 3 big boulders for this quarter?
- 3 big boulders for this month?
- 3 big boulders for this week?

If you are constantly in tune with your top three priorities, you will easily be on track to hit your 2-3 year vision. People always complain about not having enough time. They want to know how they can get more done in a day. The reason time seems problematic for most is that you don't prioritize your time. You let the day dictate where it wants to take you. When you're laser-focused on your top three priorities, or boulders, for the week, then your weeks get you to your monthly goal, which then gets you to your quarter goal, and on and on until you have realized your 2-3 year vision. With this step-by-step approach, you stop acting in desperation mode. You stop saying yes to things you know you shouldn't. Suddenly, you start to control time and bend it to your reality instead of the other way around. If you want to get your time back, master your priorities.

Congratulations! You've Made It!

The principles I teach in this book and in my coaching program are life skills, not diet skills.

I've seen clients quit their jobs and start new businesses or move out of state to align more with their true purpose. Now, you too have the blueprint for successful weight loss and for optimal health, vitality, and the mindset that will lead to success in any endeavor. You can feel comfortable in your body, in your mind, and in your path forward in life.

As famous basketball coach John Wooden once said, "I believe in the basics: attention to, and perfection of, tiny details that might be commonly overlooked. They may seem trivial, perhaps even laughable to those who don't understand, but they aren't. They are fundamental to your progress in basketball, business, and life. They are the difference between champions and near champions."

Always come back to the foundation and the fundamentals. Let your mindset and your vision ignite your passion and propel you into success in every aspect of your well-being.

Now let's go!!!!

RESOURCES

What To Do Next?

First off, I want to express my immense gratitude to you for reading this book. What lights me up and ignites my passion is knowing that if I can change just one life (you), then that person (you), will go out and impact and change someone else's life. And that person will do the same. Together, we create this crazy cycle of goodness. Imagine the change we can bring about this way! It's powerful.

That's why I say this book isn't just about weight loss. This is about transformation at the deepest level. When you're more confident and full of vitality, you'll go out and have so much impact on the world. Together, we become world-changers.

If you've come this far, it means you are a world-changer and you're dedicated to growth. Do me a favor and stay in touch. I love to connect with fellow world-changers, and I truly believe iron sharpens iron. We make each other better.

How To Stay In Touch

Over the last few years, I have learned that social media is a less reliable way to stay in touch long-term. It is prone to hacking, censorship, etc. So, based on experience, email is the best way for us to stay in touch. Go to my website **www. joelevancoaching.com** and subscribe to the email list.

Another way for us to stay connected is via my podcast, *The Hacked Life.* As of the day I'm writing this, I've done over 200 episodes, and it's growing exponentially. I'm in the process of rebranding the show to *The Joel Evan Show*, as the show has evolved beyond just health topics and biohacking. It's really become a show about higher conscious living, and teasing out what makes the best in the world phenomenal. I truly believe my podcast will be in the top five podcasts in the health and wellness category in the next 2-3 years. I've had some amazing guests already in the health, mindset, and mastery space, and it's only continuing to grow.

Lastly, if you want to work with me one-on-one, I'd love to connect. When I look back on my own life, I never would have gotten to where I'm at without mentors and teachers showing me the way to achieve my successes. Before launching my coaching business and scaling that from nothing to a six-figure business, I hired a coach because I knew nothing about creating a successful coaching business. I knew how to coach but needed to figure out how to make coaching a sustainable business. I even hired a coach when it came time to write this book. I had wanted to write a book for a while and had even purchased a course to show me the steps. Nonetheless, I hadn't taken any real action. I needed a coach, someone who had been there and done it and was already a 3x best-selling author. So I hired a coach, and it was the best money I ever spent on writing a book. He kept me on task and ensured I hit the checkpoints to succeed.

So, in my experience, every time I've invested in coaching, I've gotten so much more value out of it than the expense that I put into it. Besides results, I've gotten new ideas, new friendships, new partnerships, and so much more. If you're similarly looking to be held accountable at a high level, I'd love to connect with you and be that coach for whatever transition you're at in life.

Another Way To Be A World Changer & Work With Me

The pandemic drove so much fear and angst into the world. I saw that the stress and strain driven by Pandemic-related fear and angst were hurting people's health and well-being. People were suffering because they felt like they had very little control over so many things including their own health. I wanted to find an antidote to that fear. It struck me that understanding health on a deeper level allows people to feel more empowered.

With this in mind, I had a vision of putting a health coach in every home. Because, honestly, the more we understand true health, the more we understand ways to combat and stave off illnesses such as metabolic disease. Also, when people know the principles of health, they are able to teach and take care of one another.

It was through the work I did in trying to realize this vision that I discovered doTerra essential oils. They are one of the safest, fast-acting, effective natural remedies that I have ever found. Also, I've chosen doTerra over all other brands due to their transparency, impeccable sourcing and processing, and humanitarian efforts.

Then, if you haven't been able to tell by now, I will take things to the next level when I am certain that they are good for your health. So, rather than just using doTerra essential oils, I decided that I wanted to have a more active role with the company. To this end, I connected with doTerra's Melody Watts. She is a health mentor and a seven-figure business leader.

I am now working with Melody to build a team of mission-driven, natural health-minded individuals who want to spread this goodness, make a lot of money, and have a lot of fun. The neat thing is that I will personally mentor you along with Melody. Remember the $30k I spent to be part of Zander Fryer's Mastermind? Well, Melody and I teach the same principles and tactics discussed in my Mastermind program, but we teach our teams for free. You get this type of mentorship for free just by being one of our team members. That's how much care and value we place in our team, and we really believe we're the best and we're going to make a difference. We work with natural health practitioners that already have established businesses and help them scale to six to seven figures. We also work with people who are just starting out but who want to make a change in their family's lives and in the lives of others around them. We know that if you're WHY is big enough then anything is possible.

If you're interested in learning more about this, shoot me a message on Instagram @joelevancoaching or email me **info@joelevancoaching.com**, and I'll get you the details.

Top Biohacks For Weight Loss

Berberine

When I interviewed supplement expert and formulator Shawn Wells and asked him what would be his top five supplements if he could only choose five (this was a tough question for Shawn as he takes about 70 supplements a day), he listed berberine as one. Of his top five picks, berberine is probably the most useful supplement for weight loss because it is known as a glucose disposal agent and helps lower blood sugar levels. Berberine also has a host of other properties that make it popular for anti-aging and mitochondrial support. This is because berberine helps the body protect itself from glycation, which is a chemical reaction that results in glucose replacing protein linkages. In Shawn's book, *The Energy Formula*, he states "anti-glycation is crucial in lowering Advanced Glycation End-products (AGEs), decreasing blood glucose/HgbA1c, increasing AMPK, lowering triglycerides and inflammation and providing positive hermetic stress to mitochondria. This could be the most powerful thing I recommend when it comes to battling aging and disease and promoting wellness."

Shawn recommends taking 500 mg of berberine three times daily. Even better, 150 mg of dihydroberberine/ Glucovantage (a berberine derivative) can be taken twice daily. Dihydroberberine has been shown to be just as effective as the popular pharmaceutical drug, Metformin.

Blue Light Blocking

In order to get great, deep sleep, you need to flip on your "sleep switch." As humans, two big switches regulate our sleep. These are temperature and light. In our modern world full of artificial light, we need to regulate the light environment.

Blue-light-blocking glasses are one tool that we can use for regulating artificial light. Wearing them while looking at computer, phone and television screens for about two hours before bed can make it easier to fall asleep and stay asleep. There are several brands out there, and you can even buy them at hardware stores and on Amazon. But, these ones often look terrible and feel uncomfortable. I've been wearing TrueDark glasses as they have a red tint that blocks out the blue and green spectrums of light. It's been probably the most powerful thing to transform my sleep.

You also can change the light bulbs in your house. One way to fill your house with more sleep-conducive light is to simply buy red light bulbs on Amazon and install these in some or all of your light fixtures. However, some folks don't like their home to be lit up in all red. For my house, I have <u>Hooga Lite Bulbs</u>, which I have done in many of the rooms we use most often. These bulbs are cheap and can be found on Amazon.

BrainTap

BrainTap is a headset device that helps rewire your brain so that you can achieve better overall performance, sleep, meditation, and, even, weight loss. I'm a huge fan of this technology, especially after I interviewed Dr. Patrick Porter, the founder of BrainTap, on my podcast. He explained the way BrainTap could help rewire your subconscious. Since you know that I talked a lot about the subconscious in this book, you can imagine that I'm going to be extremely bullish on any device that can help reprogram those limiting beliefs.

When I interviewed Dr. Porter, he told me, "It's not always what you're eating that's making you gain weight, it's what's eating you. You have to change the belief in who you are. Your body doesn't give up on you, but you can give up on your body. You can't outthink a bad diet."

By some estimates, more than 80 percent of people who lose weight regain all of it back in about two years. Many people pack on even more pounds. Researchers at the University of

California at Los Angeles analyzed 31 long-term diet studies and found that about two-thirds of dieters regained more weight within four or five years than they initially lost. But, BrainTap was able to send *People Magazine* stories about 1,000 people who used their product, lost weight, and kept it off for over five years. This is huge!

CAROL Bike

As I mentioned in my exercise chapter, the CAROL bike has been a game-changer for me on those days when I can't squeeze in a workout. Being able to simulate 45 minutes of cardiovascular exercise in less than 10 minutes is powerful.

To learn more about the CAROL Bike, check out my podcast episode with the founder Ulrich Dempfle (Episode #74). You also can go to CAROL Bike's website and use the code JOELEVAN for a discount.

Cold Thermogenesis

There are many benefits to cold water immersion therapy including reducing muscle soreness, boosting immunity and improving mood. Wim Hof, known for running marathons in the cold in his swimsuit only, cites on his website that cold water immersion therapy can increase the body's metabolism by 16% and convert white fat to beneficial brown fat. Brown fat is consumed to produce heat, as opposed to unhealthy white fat which your body holds on to as an energy reserve.

In the short-term, cold exposure increases metabolism as the body has to burn calories to increase core body temperature. The total calories burned from the cold exposure are not that significant. However, when the body needs to regulate its temperature, not only is brown fat (which is highly metabolically active) activated, but white fat cells can combine with brown fat cells to create beige fat. This beige fat burns calories.

I spoke with Joshua Church, the co-founder of <u>Edge Theory Labs</u>, a company specializing in cold water therapy and making portable cold tubs. He has worked with several professional athletes and hard-charging entrepreneurs, and he believes that cold therapy is one of the best tools for developing and maintaining healthy body composition.

There are many cold tubs out there, but I'm a huge fan of the Edge Theory Labs cold tub. It's easy to set up, is portable, has a self-cleaning feature, and the water can be cooled in a matter of hours.

For more info, check out Edge Theory Labs' website and use the code JOELEVAN in checkout.

Continuous Glucose Monitor (CGM)

I've talked about glucose and insulin several times throughout this book and noted the importance of regulating glucose spikes. If glucose is elevated, insulin is generally released. Increased insulin levels lead to fat storage and weight gain.

Over time, if glucose is consistently elevated due to diet and insulin production being high, our cells can become "numb" to insulin. This is called insulin resistance, and it means that we need more and more circulating insulin to get glucose into cells. When this continues, it leads to higher baseline levels of insulin. This process will stymie anyone's weight loss efforts.

Wearing a CGM can definitely bring a higher level of awareness to your glucose and, tangentially, your insulin levels. When I interviewed Josh Clemente, founder of Levels Health, a health-based app that uses a CGM to help users make healthier eating choices, he told me he'd seen some great effects with weight loss and CGM's. As Levels Health website explains:

Real-time glucose measurements give us the power to understand how the foods we eat affect glucose levels in our blood and by rough proxy, our insulin levels. Unlike traditional dietary strategies like <u>*calorie counting*</u> *— which have been shown repeatedly to be ineffective for sustained weight loss — glucose monitoring provides insight into the underlying physiological processes that lead to fat storage.*

Josh and his team have done 28-day challenges where users that stay within a certain glucose threshold win financial prizes. He told me that the average participant loses around 10 pounds without being put on a certain diet or being told to eat specific foods.

Emotion Code

We dove deep into emotions in this book and the truth is that the way you see yourself shapes your reality. Emotions that are in disarray can lead to eating disorders, can prevent you from maintaining good habits, and can stymie your long-term growth. Remember, some trauma is passed down to us and is inherited. When you release this emotional baggage, the process becomes easier and the journey feels like less of a struggle.

For this reason, I can't recommend enough that you reach out to a good Emotion Code/Body Code practitioner. Feel free to email me at **info@joelevancoaching.com** so I can recommend a few of my favorite practitioners.

Fulvic/Humic Minerals

Scattered in several places throughout the book, I have briefly mentioned that I add fulvic minerals to my water on a daily basis. Sourced from soil and decomposed plant life, these naturally occurring minerals are typically easier for the body to digest, absorb, and utilize. I love fulvic minerals because they provide energy, and they charge to the cells to create ATP and push nutrients into the cells. They help remove toxins and heavy metals from your body, and they are good for suppressing candida yeast overgrowth and overall gut health. Humic minerals are similar but provide more of a detox effect and can help remove that pesky herbicide glyphosate that I mentioned earlier in the book. This is an absolute foundational protocol for anyone looking to get healthy.

There's a host of other reasons I'm so bullish on fulvic and humic minerals:

1. **Whole Body Systemic Effect:** Fulvic acid works on the whole body wherever it's needed — improving nerve function, weight management, and glucose balance.[35]

2. **Nutrients:** Studies suggest that when the body senses a lack of minerals and nutrition, it will develop hunger and cravings to obtain those nutrients. Using fulvic minerals can prevent that depletion from ever happening.[36]

3. **Thyroid Function:** People with a sluggish thyroid can have issues with their metabolism and the ability to lose weight. Most of the time, these folks are deficient in selenium, magnesium, zinc, and iodine. Fulvic minerals can help push those nutrients into the cells.

4. **Detoxification**: Fulvic minerals support the body with detoxification and the removal of heavy metals. This is critical since we know that our body will store toxins in fat cells.

---

35 N. A. Trivedi, B. Mazumdar, J. D. Bhatt, and K. G. Hemavathi, "Effect of shilajit on blood glucose and lipid profile in alloxan-induced diabetic rats," *Indian Journal of Pharmacology 36,* no. 6 (December 2004): 373–376, http://www.bioline.org.br/pdf?ph04132.

36 Katherine Harmon, "Addicted to Fat: Overeating May Alter the Brain as Much as Hard Drugs," *Scientific American,* March 28, 2010, https://www.scientificamerican.com/article/addicted-to-fat-eating/.

5. **Diabetes**: Traditional medicine and modern research show that fulvic minerals can improve some of the problems that are hallmarks of diabetes. Fulvic minerals help modulate the immune system, influence the oxidative state of cells, and improve gastrointestinal function.[37]

To learn more about fulvic/humic minerals, check out my **podcast** with Caroline Alan (Episode #174) from **BEAM Minerals** (use code JOELEVAN for a discount). Caroline had a host of health issues, and, just by taking fulvic minerals, she was able to restore her health.

Infrared Sauna

I'm a huge fan of saunas and have repeatedly said on my podcast that it's probably the best pound-for-pound biohack you can get for the money. I prefer infrared saunas over dry heat saunas since infrared rays heat deeper layers of the body at lower temperatures than the warm air associated with traditional saunas. This provokes a more efficient sweat response. A full-spectrum infrared sauna will deliver the cardiovascular requirements the body needs to maintain its internal core temperature (a process known as homeostasis) because one session in an infrared sauna is akin to a moderately-paced walk or light jog. You're essentially stimulating exercise by being in an infrared sauna. A 2017 study in the European

---

37 John Winkler and Sanjoy Ghosh, "Therapeutic Potential of Fulvic Acid in Chronic Inflammatory Diseases and Diabetes," *Journal of Diabetes Research* (September 2018): 5391014, https://doi.org/10.1155/2018/5391014.

Journal of Preventive Cardiology discovered that infrared sauna users maintained an elevated heart rate for about 30 minutes after one sauna session. On top of improving your cardiovascular health, infrared saunas also promote detox which, as we know, is critical since toxins like to hide out in fat cells.

Amongst the above listed benefits, what about sauna and weight loss? Let's explore a couple ideas. First, saunas have been shown to increase growth hormone dramatically, and as learned earlier in the book, growth hormone has a profound effect in lipolysis, the breakdown of body fat. A study of seventeen men and women who were exposed to two one-hour sauna sessions at 80°C (176°F) dry heat (typical Finnish-style sauna) per day for seven days exhibited a 16-fold increase in growth hormone levels by the third day.[38] Secondly, saunas seem to have an effect on insulin sensitivity. We learned earlier in the book the importance of managing your insulin levels as when these levels become out of range, we see a host of metabolic disorders such as diabetes, cardiovascular disease, high cholesterol, high blood pressure, and of course, weight gain. Repeated treatment with a far-infrared sauna has been shown to significantly lower fasting

---

38   J. Leppäluoto, P. Huttunen, J. Hirvonen, A. Väänänen, M. Tuominen, and J. Vuori, "Endocrine effects of repeated sauna bathing," *Acta Physiologica Scandinavica 128,* no. 3 (November 1986): 467–470, https://doi.org/10.1111/j.1748-1716.1986.tb08000.x.

blood glucose levels.[39] When insulin resistant diabetic mice were subjected to 30 minutes of heat treatment three times a week for 12 weeks, they experienced a 31 percent decrease in plasma insulin levels and a significant reduction in blood glucose levels, suggesting re-sensitization to insulin.[40] Lastly, by increasing your heart rate and metabolism, you'll burn calories. All of this is why I see infrared saunas as a great tool for aiding in weight loss.

My personal favorite infrared sauna is the Therasage. It's portable and allows me to multi-task and work while I'm inside the sauna because my hands can be free. In addition to providing infrared rays, the Therasage also includes red light photobiomodulation, which is good for reducing inflammation and pain, and a grounding plate. I've had a chance to speak with Robby Besner, the owner of Therasage, and he's just a terrific man with a huge heart who wants to change the world. He also takes a lot of pride in his work and uses a lot of care when crafting his products. Robbie was gracious enough to give my audience a discount code. Use the code JOELEVAN in checkout.

---

39 Masakazu Imamura MD et al., "Repeated thermal therapy improves impaired vascular endothelial function in patients with coronary risk factors," *Journal of the American College of Cardiology 38,* no. 4 (October 2001): 1083–1088, https://doi.org/10.1016/S0735-1097(01)01467-X.

40 Satoshi Kokura et al., "Whole body hypothermia improves obesity-induced insulin resistance in diabetic mice," *International Journal of Hyperthermia 23,* no. 3 (2007): 259–265, https://doi.org/10.1080/02656730601176824.

LeelaQ Tech Frequency Cards

LeelaQ Tech makes a frequency card that you can simply put in your pocket that helps reduce cravings, increase metabolism, and to make it easier to follow through with efforts to manage weight on a mental and physical level. This sounds quite woo-woo that a frequency card you put in your pocket or have on your person could help you lose weight. Personally, I've never used the frequency card for weight loss, but I do vouch for LeelaQ Tech's products, as I've had a chance to sit down with the founder several times and discuss the science behind his products. I also own several of his other products such as Infinity Bloc, capsules, and Inner Peace Frequency Card, where I have noticed differences between me and my household. Besides my testimony, LeelaQ Tech has had several third-party tests such as live bloody analyses, dark field microscopy, advanced Deka Voll methods by the Besa Institute, Bio-Well (registered medical diagnosis device in Europe and Russia), EMF meter testing for all clothing products, and Emoto Institute's water crystal analyses. All the various third-party tests showed significant differences before and after a person was without LeelaQ Tech and then after when they were exposed to the tech. Here's the deal, we are beings of frequency. Everything is energy. Most of us are in tune with the wrong energy or are attracting frequencies limiting us. I've found that when you're in tune with the right frequency, everything gets easier. As my mentor, David Meltzer says, "Your frequency is your neighborhood."

MetaPWR

I've been using essential oils for about 9 years now since the birth of my first child. I've always found them effective, but the last six months I've really been geeking out on them and taking a deep dive with many experts. Also, interestingly enough, there are some essential oils that can be beneficial for metabolic health.

doTerra's MetaPWR Metabolic Blend features proprietary balanced ratios of several essential oils: Grapefruit, Lemon, Peppermint, Ginger, and Cinnamon Bark. Preclinical research suggests Grapefruit, with its naturally high levels of the chemical constituent limonene, may support a healthy metabolism when ingested. Lemon is also high in limonene. The Peppermint ingredient in MetaPWR supports weight loss efforts by curbing hunger cravings between meals. Other recent preclinical research on the MetaPWR essential oil blend suggests that it can limit the development of new fat cells and the growth of existing fat cells. Grapefruit oil, specifically, is known for preventing the maturation or growth of fat cells. Cinnamon bark is also great for helping blunt blood glucose spikes.

In addition, you can find both berberine and mulberry leaf extract in doTerra's MetaPWR Assist capsules.

Mulberry Leaf Extract

Mulberry leaf extract has been shown to reduce carbohydrate digestion by 42% when taken with a meal. Basically, it slows down the conversion of carbohydrates to glucose (blood sugar), so, instead of a giant spike and then drop in your blood sugar levels, your blood sugar stays within a more optimal curve. Similar to berberine, mulberry leaf extract has shown some promising features.[41]

Neubie by Neufit

The Neubie device is like nothing else you've seen. Created by Garrett Salpeter and his team at Neufit, the Neubie is FDA-cleared* and patented. It safely sends direct current signals to precisely where you are experiencing pain or muscle movement limitations. These signals re-educate your muscles by tapping into the power of the nervous system. The Neubie can be used for reduction in pain/inflammation, for help with neurological disorders, and for promoting muscle growth/hypertrophy.

If any of you already follow me, then you know that the Neubie device is one of my favorite biohacks. In fact, it is one of the most effective all-around technologies I know. Back in 2017, I met

---

41 Mark Lown et al., "Mulberry-extract improves glucose tolerance and decreases insulin concentrations in normoglycaemic adults: Results of a randomised double-blind placebo-controlled study," *PLoS One 12,* no. 2 (February 2017): e0172239, https://doi.org/10.1371/journal.pone.0172239.

Garrett and saw what the Neubie could do. I was so enthralled with it that I later flew out to Texas to get trained on how to use the device so that I could help others in my local area.

But, how is the Neubie beneficial for weight loss?

First, and perhaps surprisingly, the Neubie helps with something known as the 'Master Reset.' The Master Reset occurs when direct current is run all throughout the body thereby causing the nervous system to reset into a parasympathetic state and heart rate variability (HRV) is increased. As a result, you become more relaxed. When we looked at cortisol in the chapter on exercise, we saw that excessive stress hormones can ruin body composition. Being more relaxed allows our hormones to be more balanced. Just look at what happens to men when they go on TRT, for example, after being testosterone-depleted for many years. This is anecdotal, but it makes sense. If we can lower stress and improve recovery, that's naturally going to have a positive effect on body composition.

Second, Neufit has conducted some good studies with their device on hypertrophy and building muscle. The Neubie can create muscle-building benefits that are similar to traditional high-resistance exercise. Truthfully, it can pulse your muscles more times per second and create more metabolic demand and fatigue than any amount of weights could ever create. Of course, greater muscle mass is helpful for regulating blood sugar and improving hormones as well.

Lastly, and this is anectodal and more observational, when training with the Neubie many people report an elevated metabolic rate, and for longer duration. Just like with effective HIIT, you can get an additional metabolic boost for many hours after training.

For more information on the Neubie device, check out my podcast with the founder, Garret Salpeter (Episode #61).

Pendulum Glucose Control

Gut health is very important, and probiotics help improve the gut microbiome. I interviewed Coleen Cutcliffe, co-founder of Pendulum, which is a company that produces several probiotic products. I was fascinated to learn how much of a role the gut microbiome plays in regulating glucose and diabetes. Pendulum's flagship product *Glucose Control*, a blend of *Akkermansia muciniphila* and four other high-potency bacterial strains, has been shown to help lower A1C and post-meal glucose spikes in people with Type 2 diabetes who are also taking Metformin. People with Type 2 diabetes are shown to be deficient in Akkermansia, which is associated with healthy weight management. In a double-blind, placebo-controlled nutrition study, *Pendulum's Glucose Control* was demonstrated to drop A1C by -0.6%, and it reduced post-prandial glucose spikes by 32.5%.[42]

---

42 Fanny Perraudeau et. al., "Improvements to postprandial glucose control in subjects with type 2 diabetes: a multicenter, double blind, randomized placebo-controlled trial of a novel probiotic formulation," *BJM Open Diabetes Research and Care,* no. 8 (July 2020): e001319, https://doi.org/10.1136/bmjdrc-2020-001319.

Pendulum's precise anaerobic strains also restore the body's natural capability to produce the postbiotic butyrate. Postbiotics are the healthy by-products of digestion in a well-balanced gut, and butyrate is a postbiotic that binds to specific receptors within the gut mucosa and stimulates the release of glucagon-like peptide-1 (GLP-1) which, in turn, stimulates insulin secretion. GLP-1 is deficient in people with impaired glucose tolerance and Type 2 diabetes, and this contributes to hyperglycemia.

The benefits of GLP-1 go beyond diabetes. Balancing blood sugar is vital to health. In people who are not living with Type 2 diabetes, GLP-1:

- Promotes satiety and reduces appetite
- Improves glucose control
- Boosts metabolic health

Having a healthy gut microbiome is critical for overall health, and taking this probiotic would be healthy for someone even if they didn't have weight management issues.

For more information about Pendulum's *Glucose Control*, check out my podcast with Coleen (Episode #183).

Also, if you go to Pendulum's website, you can use the code HACKED for a discount.

Red Light Therapy (RLT) and Near-Infrared (NIR)

Both RLT, which is red light that you can see, and NIR, which you cannot see but you can feel as heat, are known to promote healing. They work by increasing circulation and lowering inflammation. So, although there's not a ton of research to suggest that these therapies directly lead to fat loss, these therapies do have a positive impact on problems that affect people suffering from weight loss issues. Also, at a cellular level, red/near-infrared light can elicit a response that causes fat cells to release stored fat into the bloodstream. Once in the circulatory system, the fat can then be burned off as energy. Conveniently, this can be accomplished without compromising blood serum lipid profiles. One study showed that this fat loss could be significantly amplified when combined with a regular exercise regimen. A group of 20 women riding stationary bicycles three times per week for four weeks while being exposed to near-infrared (NIR) lost an average of 444% more fat compared to 20 women doing the same exercise without NIR.[43]

When I spoke with Scott Kennedy, owner of Lightpath, a RLT company, he told me that he believes RLT can help with weight loss for other reasons. RLT improves recovery and heart rate variability, and it helps place the body in a more parasympathetic or rested/relaxed state. This all leads to better overall balance in the body, improved sleep, and

---

43 Frank Möckel, Gerd Hoffmann, Roy Overmüller, Wolfgang Drobnik, and Gerd Schmitz, "Influence of water-filtered infrared-A (wIRA) on reduction of local fat and body weight by physical exercise," *GMS German Medical Science,* no. 4 (July 2006), https://www.ncbi.nlm.nih.gov/pmc/articles/PMC2703221/.

improved digestion. These downstream effects would then promote overall weight loss.

To learn more about Scott and some of the great work he's doing over at Lightpath, go to **https://lightpathled.com/**

Semaglutide

Semaglutide is part of the class of medications called GLP-1 receptor agonists or glucagon-like peptide-1 receptor agonists that I explained in the Pendulum Glucose Control section. It increases insulin secretion, which is good for diabetes. But, at higher doses, it acts on centers in the brain and suppresses appetite. When I interviewed Josh Whalen, the CEO of Blokes Modern Men's Health and Joi Women's Wellness, he told me they were successfully administering this peptide to their users all across the United States and seeing magnificent results in long-term weight loss. One of the biggest reasons people can't lose weight long-term is their difficulty managing their appetite. Semaglutide helps regulate appetite. When people were administered 2.4 mg of subcutaneous semaglutide weekly and coupled this with lifestyle changes, the **results were a mean 10% to 15% weight loss** (10 to 15 kg) over 68 weeks versus 2% to 3% (3 to 4 kg) with placebo (PC). Most people (70% to 80%) lost 5% or more of their body weight. About 75% had gastrointestinal side effects, but few discontinued treatments as a result.[44] That's a big deal.

---

44   John P.H. Wilding et al., "Once-Weekly Semaglutide in Adults with Overweight or Obesity," *New England Journal of Medicine 384,* no. 11 (March 2021): 989–1002, https://doi.org/10.1056/NEJMoa2032183.

To learn more about Josh and his team, go to **blokes.co**. You also can check out my **podcast** with Josh (Episode #112).

Sleepme or Eight Sleep

We know the importance of sleep and how it impacts recovery, improves your brain's decision-making capacity, and helps regulate the hormones that affect appetite. Getting more sleep and deeper sleep seems to be the most beneficial thing we can do for the body in terms of overall recovery. A nice hack for getting into deep sleep faster and staying asleep longer is by controlling body temperature. Using technologies like the Eight Sleep mattress or the Sleepme mattress topper to cool your body to a specific temperature throughout the night can be very beneficial.

Scan the QR code below to get a links and discounts to all the resources I listed.

Acknowledgements

This book is a testament to the giants whose shoulders I stand upon. Thank you to my wife Nini for always seeing my blind spots and making me strive to be better. Thank you to my mom for always supporting me, even when we didn't see eye to eye, you've always loved and supported my dreams. This book could not have happened without your support over the last two years. Thanks to my pops for always providing unconditional love and support and instilling in me at an early age the "Rocky mentality." Thank you David Amiccuci for teaching me to strike first, strike fast, and never give up (I'm still on a quest to be my best, TRK). Carlos Sapao, thank you for your support and for helping me name this book. Thank you to my brother Adam, for always supporting me and sharpening my sword in the ways others cannot. Thank you Sean O'Keefe for loving me like a brother and supporting me since I was a young buck, Cutco salesman. I'm still No Limit. Thank you Jake Kelfer for pushing me to write this book at record speed and holding me accountable to make this book a bestseller. Thank you George and Melissa Ryan for your endless support, when the rest of the world shunned me, you embraced me.

Made in the USA
Thornton, CO
06/08/24 08:40:53

cd46f07c-5cb7-4a2f-afeb-e1944bde816eR01